MYLES MIDWIFERY

ANATOMY AND PHYSIOLOGY
WORKBOOK

This book is dedicated to my young nephew, David Porter (1991–2009)

Illic est usquequaque soles secundum pluvial.

Content Strategist: Mairi McCubbin
Content Development Specialist: Sheila Black
Project Manager: Julie Taylor
Designer: Kirsteen Wright and Miles Hitchen
Illustration Manager: Jennifer Rose
Illustrators: Amanda Williams and Ian Ramsden; adapted by Antbits Ltd

MYLES MIDWIFERY

ANATOMY AND PHYSIOLOGY WORKBOOK

Jean Rankin BSc(Hons) MSc PhD PGCE RM RGN RSCN
Lead Midwife for Education, School of Health, Nursing and Midwifery,
University of the West of Scotland, Paisley; Supervisor of Midwives – Ayrshire and Arran, UK

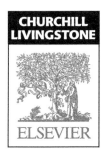

CHURCHILL LIVINGSTONE

ELSEVIER

Edinburgh   London   New York   Oxford   Philadelphia   St Louis   Sydney   Toronto   2013

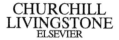

CHURCHILL
LIVINGSTONE
ELSEVIER

ISBN 978-0-7020-4339-0
Reprinted 2013, 2014, 2017 (twice)

British Library Cataloguing in Publication Data
A catalogue record for this book is available from the British Library

Library of Congress Cataloging in Publication Data
A catalog record for this book is available from the Library of Congress

Notices
Knowledge and best practice in this field are constantly changing. As new research and experience broaden our understanding, changes in research methods, professional practices, or medical treatment may become necessary.

Practitioners and researchers must always rely on their own experience and knowledge in evaluating and using any information, methods, compounds, or experiments described herein. In using such information or methods they should be mindful of their own safety and the safety of others, including parties for whom they have a professional responsibility.

With respect to any drug or pharmaceutical products identified, readers are advised to check the most current information provided (i) on procedures featured or (ii) by the manufacturer of each product to be administered, to verify the recommended dose or formula, the method and duration of administration, and contraindications. It is the responsibility of practitioners, relying on their own experience and knowledge of their patients, to make diagnoses, to determine dosages and the best treatment for each individual patient, and to take all appropriate safety precautions.

To the fullest extent of the law, neither the Publisher nor the authors, contributors, or editors, assume any liability for any injury and/or damage to persons or property as a matter of products liability, negligence or otherwise, or from any use or operation of any methods, products, instructions, or ideas contained in the material herein.

ELSEVIER your source for books, journals and multimedia in the health sciences
www.elsevierhealth.com

Working together to grow libraries in developing countries
www.elsevier.com | www.bookaid.org | www.sabre.org

ELSEVIER   BOOK AID International   Sabre Foundation

The publisher's policy is to use paper manufactured from sustainable forests

Printed in Great Britain
Last digit is the print number: 15 14 13 12 11 10 9 8

Contents

How to use this book
Icons and activities

This anatomy and physiology activity book is aimed at student midwives. The purpose is to provide a range of activities to assist them in the revision of their knowledge related to pregnancy, labour, childbirth, puerperium and the neonate. The sections of the book closely follow the anatomy and physiology sections of the relevant chapters in the current *Myles Textbook for Midwives* (2009) and relevant national guidelines (where appropriate).

Word lists and labels are provided with a number of the activities to prompt and guide students as they complete the activities. Students should refer to the textbook when completing those activities where no prompts are provided.

 Colouring: identify and colour structures on diagrams

 Labelling: identify and label structures on diagrams

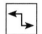 **Matching:** match statements in a variety of ways, e.g. structures with functions; structures with conditions; key choices with blanks in a paragraph, etc.

Combinations of these activities are also used to provide variety in the text for students.

 Completion: identify the missing word(s) or remove incorrect word(s) to complete activities – when completing then students should carefully consider the information required to ensure the correct information is provided.

 True/false: Students are required to identify if statements are true or false. Again, these should be carefully considered and not be assumed to be correct. If the statement chosen is incorrect or false then the student should refer to the textbook or relevant national guidelines for the correct response.

 Short answers: Students are required to refer to the textbook and provide short answers to complete the activities.

 Definitions: explain the meaning of common obstetric, midwifery, neonatal terminology and anatomical and physiological terms.

 Multiple choice questions: identify the correct answer from the list of four or five options. There is only one correct response for each MCQ.

 Pot luck: a small number of activities are labelled 'pot luck' as they bring together a range of different topics within the same section.

Acknowledgements

Special thanks to Lyz Howie, Midwife Lecturer at the University of the West of Scotland, for her advice and support.

1 The female pelvis and pelvic floor

Midwives need to have sound knowledge of the anatomy of the normal female pelvis. It is one of the ways to estimate a woman's progress in labour by assessing the relationship of the fetus to certain pelvic landmarks. Knowledge of pelvic anatomy is also essential to detect deviations from normal. The activities in this chapter will test your knowledge of the related topics.

THE PELVIC GIRDLE

The pelvic bones

 Completion

1. The pelvic girdle is composed of four bones: two innominate bones, the sacrum and coccyx. Each innominate bone is made up of three bones that have fused together: the ilium, the ischium and the pubis. Decide where the following statements apply to the bones of the pelvic girdle and complete Table 1.1 by ticking the appropriate column(s).

Table 1.1

Descriptive statement	Ilium	Ischium	Sacrum	Coccyx
a. It is the thick lower part				
b. It is the wedge-shaped bone				
c. The upper border is the iliac crest				
d. The anterior surface is concave and referred to as the hollow				
e. It has a large prominence known as the ischial tuberosity				
f. It consists of four fused vertebrae				
g. The pubis forms the anterior part				
h. It is a vestigial tail				
i. The upper border of the first vertebra of this bone juts forward and is known as the promontory				
j. The concave anterior surface is the iliac fossa				
k. The ischial spines are located here				
l. It consists of five fused vertebrae				
m. The posterior surface is roughened to receive muscle attachments				
n. It is the large flared-out part				
o. Laterally the bone extends into a wing or ala				
p. The bone is pierced with four pairs of foramina through which nerves emerge to supply the pelvic organs				

 Labelling

2. Figure 1.1 shows the pelvic bones. Label the four bones of the pelvic girdle and label the symphysis pubis.

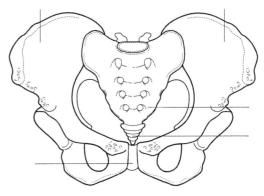

Figure 1.1

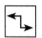 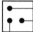 ## Matching and labelling

3. Figure 1. 2 shows the lateral view of the innominate bone. The innominate bone contains a deep cup termed the acetabulum which receives the head of the femur. The acetabulum is composed of three fused bones (two-fifths ilium, two-fifths ischium and one-fifth pubis). Label the detailed landmarks of the innominate bone by matching to the key choices listed below.

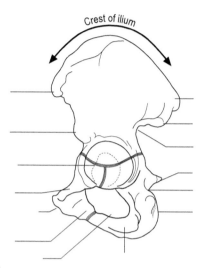

Posterior superior iliac spine
Acetabulum
Superior ramus of pubic bone
Anterior inferior iliac spine
Lesser sciatic notch
Ischial tuberosity
Inferior ramus of ischium
Anterior superior iliac spine
Symphysis pubis
Ischial spine
Obturator foramen
Posterior inferior iliac spine
Inferior ramus of pubic bone
Greater sciatic notch

Figure 1.2

Pelvic joints and ligaments

 ## Completion

4. There are four pelvic joints: one sacrococcygeal joint, one symphysis pubis joint and two sacroiliac joints. Complete the following sentences from the key words below (some words may be used more than once).

Base   Pelvis   Sacrum   Rami   Left   Right

Pubic bones   Ilium   Spine   Tip   Coccyx

1. The **symphysis pubis** is the midline cartilaginous joint uniting the _____ of the _____ and _____

   _____.

2. The **sacroiliac joints** join the _____ to the _____ and as a result connect the _____ to

   the _____.

3. The **sacrococcygeal joint** is formed where the _____ of the _____ articulates with the

   _____ of the sacrum.

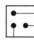 ## Matching, colouring and labelling

5. Figure 1.3 provides a posterior view of the pelvis showing the ligaments. Label and colour the appropriate landmarks and ligaments by matching to the key choices provided below.

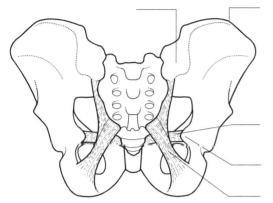

Ischial spine
Iliac crest
Posterior superior iliac spine
Sacrospinal ligament
Sacrotuberous ligament

Figure 1.3

Types of pelvis

 ## Labelling

6. There are four categories of pelves: gynaecoid, android, anthropoid and platypelloid. Label the following categories of pelves in Figure 1.4.

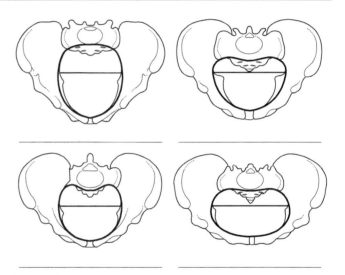

Figure 1.4

 ## Completion

7. Consider the descriptive words provided below. Complete Table 1.2 by choosing the words most appropriate to describe the features of the different types of pelvis (some words may be used more than once).

Kidney-shaped	Narrow	Generous	Heart-shaped
Rounded	Narrowed	Convergent	Divergent
Long oval	Wide	Straight	

Table 1.2

Features	Gynaecoid	Anthropoid	Platypelloid	Android
Brim				
Forepelvis				
Side walls				

Labelling

8. Label the features of the gynaecoid pelvis shown in Figure 1.5. Beside each label use a descriptive term to indicate why this pelvis is suitable for childbirth (e.g. cavity shallow, outlet wide, etc.).

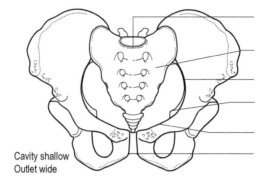

Cavity shallow
Outlet wide

Figure 1.5

 Completion

9. Table 1.3 provides statements related to the pelves. Complete the table by correctly matching the statements to the appropriate type of pelves by ticking the relevant box(es). Some statements may relate to more than one pelvis.

Table 1.3

Statement	Gynaecoid	Android	Anthropoid	Platypelloid
a. It has straight side walls and a shallow cavity				
b. The anteroposterior diameter is reduced and the transverse diameter increased				
c. Its brim is heart-shaped				
d. The side walls converge making it funnel-shaped				
e. There is a long oval brim				
f. It has a rounded brim and a sub-pubic arch of 90°				
g. It has a narrow forepelvis				
h. It has a kidney-shaped brim				
i. It has a deep cavity and straight sacrum				
j. The sub-pubic arch is <90°				
k. It has a generous forepelvis				
l. The side walls diverge				
m. The anteroposterior diameter is longer than the transverse diameter				
n. The transverse diameter is situated towards the back				
o. The sacrum is long and deeply concave				
p. The sacrum is flat and the cavity shallow				
q. The sub-pubic angle is wide (>90°)				
r. The ischial spines are prominent				
s. It has a well-curved sacrum				
t. The ischial spines are blunt and not prominent in these pelves				
u. The forepelvis is narrow with the greater space found in the hindpelvis				

The pelvis in relation to pregnancy and childbirth

 Definitions

10. The pelvis is divided into the true and false pelvis. Complete the following definitions from the extended list of words provided below (words may be used more than once):

Fetus	Bony canal	Brim	Pubic bones	Baby
Flared-out	Ischial tuberosities	Sacral promontory	Lower	Cavity
Above	Curve of Carus	Iliac	Ischial	Abdominal
Lateral	Upper	Pelvic	Below	Birth
Outlet				

1. The true pelvis is the _____ through which the _____ must pass

    during _____.

2. The true pelvis is divided into three components: a. _____ _____, b. _____

    _____, c. _____ _____.

3. The false pelvis is the part of the pelvis which is situated _____ the _____

    _____. It is formed by the _____ _____ portions of the _____

    bones and protects the _____ organs.

The true pelvis

 Matching and labelling

11. The superior circumference forms the pelvic brim with the included space called the inlet. Figure 1.6 shows the brim of the female pelvis. Match the landmarks a–h with the list provided. In addition insert and label the sacrocotyloid dimension.

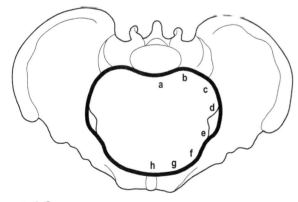

Figure 1.6

Iliopectineal line: _____

Sacral promontory: _____

Sacroiliac joint: _____

Superior ramus of the pubic border: _____

Sacral ala or wing: _____

Upper inner border of the symphysis pubis: _____

Iliopectineal eminence: _____

Upper inner border of the pubic bone: _____

Pelvic diameters

It is essential that practising midwives have knowledge of the pelvic diameters of the normal pelvis. Contraction of any of the diameters can result in malposition or malpresentation of the presenting part of the fetus.

  ## Matching and labelling

12. Figure 1.7 provides a view of the pelvic brim showing diameters. Label the diameters of the pelvic brim by matching to the key below.

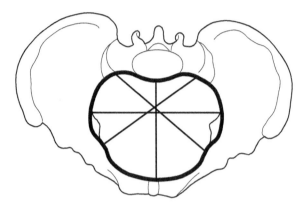

Transverse
Left oblique
Right oblique
Anteroposterior

Figure 1.7

 ## Completion

13. Complete the following statements about pelvic brim diameters by choosing the correct key words (11 in total) taken from the extended list of pelvis-related words below.

Greatest width	Symphysis	Sacrum	Brim
Iliopectineal	Conjugate	Sacroiliac	Smallest width
Sacral	Cavity	Outlet	Ischial spines
Pubis	Promontory	Eminence	Iliac

1. The transverse diameter extends across the _____ of the _____.

2. The oblique diameter extends from the _____ _____ of one side to the

    _____ articulation of the opposite side.

3. The anteroposterior diameter extends from the _____ _____

    to the _____ _____. The other term for this diameter is the

    _____ diameter.

Completion

14. Insert the correct measurement for each of the diameters (cm) of the pelvic brim, cavity and outlet in Figure 1.8.

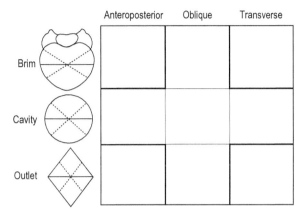

Figure 1.8

Conjugate diameters

Three conjugate diameters can be measured: anatomical conjugate, obstetric conjugate and diagonal conjugate. Two of these diameters may be referred to as the 'true' conjugate. Therefore the midwife must be aware of this fact and be clear as to the conjugate measurement being referred to in any situation.

 Completion

15. Consider the following statements and decide where they apply to the conjugate diameters. Complete Table 1.4 by ticking in the appropriate column(s).

Table 1.4

Statement	Anatomical conjugate	Obstetrical conjugate	Diagonal (Internal) conjugate
a. Measurement averages 12 cm			
b. Is measured from the sacral promontory to the posterior border of the upper surface of the symphysis pubis			
c. Is measured anteroposteriorly from the lower border of the symphysis to the sacral promontory			
d. Is measured from the sacral promontory to the uppermost point of the symphysis pubis			
e. Measurement averages 11 cm			
f. This conjugate is of significance to midwives			
g. This measurement is not assessed in the UK			
h. Measurement averages 12–13 cm			
i. This measurement represents the available space for the passage of the fetal head through the bony pelvis			
j. The term true conjugate may be used to refer to these two conjugate diameters			

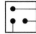 **Matching and labelling**

16. Figure 1.9 represents the median section of the pelvis showing anteroposterior diameters. Label the following figure by matching to the key provided.

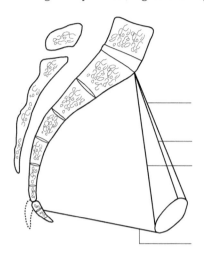

Figure 1.9

Obstetrical conjugate
Internal or diagonal conjugate
Obstetrical anterior of outlet
Anatomical conjugate (true)
Anteroposterior of outlet

Asynclitism

 Completion

17. Think carefully about how the fetal head negotiates the pelvic brim and then complete the following section using the relevant key words from the extended list below (some words may be used more than once).

Anterior	Head	External	Parietal eminence
Flexion	Internal	Symphysis pubis	Lateral
Sacral promontory	Reversed	Posterior	Similar
Oblique	Opposite	Rotation	Anteroposterior
Ischial spines	Ischial tuberosity	Biparietal	Sacral hollow
Posterior	Descent	Rotation	
Cavity	Same	Outlet	

1. Engagement may necessitate _____ tilting of the head, known as asynclitism, in order to

    allow the _____ diameter to pass the narrowest _____ diameter of

    the brim.

2. In anterior asynclitism, the _____ parietal bone moves down behind the

    _____ until the _____ enters the brim. The movement

    is then reversed and the head tilts in the _____ direction until the _____

    parietal bone negotiates the _____ and the head is engaged.

3. In posterior asynclitism, the movements of anterior asynclitism are _____.

The _____ parietal bone negotiates the _____ prior to the

_____ parietal bone moving down behind the _____. Once

the pelvic brim has been negotiated, _____ progresses normally accompanied by

_____ and _____ rotation.

Miscellaneous questions about the pelvis

True/false

18. Consider the following statements and choose if they are true or false by ticking the appropriate column.

	Statement	True	False
a.	The anterior superior iliac spine is the bony prominences felt at the back of the iliac crests		
b.	The concave posterior surface of the ilium is the iliac fossa		
c.	The lesser sciatic notch lies between the ischial spine and ischial tuberosity		
d.	The sacrococcygeal joint permits the coccyx to be deflected forwards during the birth of the fetal head		
e.	The obstetrical outlet is of greater practical significance because it includes the narrow pelvic strait through which the fetus must pass		
f.	The obturator foramen is the space enclosed by the body of the pubic bone, the rami and the ileum		
g.	Sacrocotyloid dimension passes from the sacral promontory to the iliopectineal eminence on each side and measures 12 cm		
h.	A widening of 1–2 cm at the symphysis pubis during pregnancy above the normal gap of 7–8 cm is normal		
i.	The obstetrical outlet is the space between the narrow pelvic strait and the anatomical outlet		
j.	In the standing position, the pelvis is placed such that the anterior superior iliac spine and the front edge of the symphysis pubis are in the same vertical plane, perpendicular to the floor		
k.	Structures passing through the pelvic brim never affect the space available for the fetus, for instance, the descending colon enters the pelvis near the right sacroiliac joint		
l.	A line drawn exactly half-way between the lateral walls of the pelvic canal would trace a curve known as the curve of Carus		
m.	The <u>obstetrical</u> conjugate is measured from the sacral promontory to the posterior border of the upper surface of the symphysis pubis (1.25 cm lower). Measurement averages 11 cm		
n.	The height of the individual influences the size of the pelvis and in general, women of short stature tend to have narrow pelves		
o.	The sacroiliac joints are strong non-weight-bearing synovial joints		
p.	High assimilation pelvis occurs when the 5th lumbar vertebra is fused to the sacrum and the angle of inclination of the pelvic brim is increased		
q.	The sacrotuberous ligaments and sacrospinous ligaments pass between the sacrum and ischium		
r.	The narrow pelvic strait lies between the sacrococcygeal joint, the two ischial spines and the upper border of the symphysis pubis		

? Multiple choice questions (MCQs)

19. Consider each of the following statements and choose the correct answer(s) to complete the statements.

1. If the line joining the sacral promontory and the top of the symphysis pubis were extended then the angle

   formed with the horizontal floor would be _____:

   a. 60°   b. 90°   c. 45°

2. The pelvic girdle is a _____:

   a. funnel-shaped cavity   b. basin-shaped cavity   c. heart-shaped cavity

3. The greater sciatic notch is a curve extending from the posterior iliac spine to the _____:

   a. ischial spine   b. ischial tuberosity   c. pubic bones

4. The depth of the anterior wall of the cavity is _____:

   a. 4 cm   b. 6 cm   c. 10 cm

5. The length of the posterior wall of the cavity is _____:

   a. 6 cm   b. 10 cm   c. 12 cm

6. The sacrocotyloid dimension passes from the sacral promontory to the iliopectineal eminence on each side

   and measures _____:

   a. 9–9.5 cm   b. 10 cm   c. 11 cm

7. The sub-pubic angle of the platypelloid pelvis is _____:

   a. Less than 90°   b. 90°   c. Greater than 90°

8. The incidence of women with an android pelvis is reported to be _____:

   a. 50%   b. 20%   c. 25%

20. Consider the following statements.

1. Choose the correct answer(s):

   a. In the justo minor pelvis all pelvic diameters can be 1.25 cm smaller than average.

   b. The pelvis is said to be contracted if one of the diameters is smaller than normal by 2 cm or more.

   c. The anterior wall of the cavity is formed by the curve of the sacrum and is 12 cm in length.

   d. All of the above.

   e. None of the above.

2. Choose the correct answer(s):

   a. The ischial tuberosity is a bony prominence found on the ilium.

   b. The lateral walls of the outlet are mainly covered by the obturator internus muscles.

   c. The anatomical outlet is formed by the upper borders of each of the bones together with the sacrotuberous ligament.

   d. None of the above.

   e. All of the above.

3. Choose the correct answer(s):

   a. The anatomical outlet is formed by the lower borders of each of the bones together with the sacrotuberous ligament.

   b. The ischial tuberosity is a bony prominence found on the ischium.

   c. The sacrocotyloid dimension is important with posterior positions of the occiput when the parietal eminences of the fetal head may become caught.

   d. All of the above.

   e. None of the above.

4. Choose the correct answer(s):

   a. In posterior positions of the occiput it is the sacrocotyloid dimension that becomes important as the parietal eminences of the fetal head may become caught.

   b. In the standing position the pelvis is placed such that the anterior superior iliac spine and the front edge of the symphysis pubis are in the same vertical plane.

   c. Pelvic planes are imaginary flat surfaces at the brim, cavity and outlet of the pelvic canal.

   d. None of the above.

   e. All of the above.

Deformed pelves

 Short answers

21. Deformed pelves may occur for a variety of reasons including developmental anomaly, dietary deficiency, injury or disease. Complete the following sections about the different causes of deformed pelves.

   1. Dietary deficiency

   Give **one** example and describe the deformity:

   Example: _____

   a. Describe the condition: _____

   _____

   _____

   b. Describe the general effect of the condition on the pelvis: _____

   _____

   _____

   c. Relate the deformity/abnormality of the pelvis to childbirth: _____

   _____

   _____

2. Developmental anomalies

Give **one** example and describe the anomaly:

Example: _____

    a. Describe the condition: _____

    _____

    _____

    b. Describe the general effect of the condition on the pelvis: _____

    _____

    c. Relate the deformity/abnormality of the pelvis to childbirth: _____

    _____

3. Injury and disease

Give **one** example and describe the deformity:

Example: _____

    a. Describe the condition: _____

    _____

    b. Describe the general effect of the condition on the pelvis: _____

    _____

    _____

THE PELVIC FLOOR

Functions of the pelvic floor

The pelvic floor is formed by the soft tissues that fill the outlet of the pelvis. The most important of these is the strong diaphragm of muscle slung like a hammock from the walls of the pelvis. The urethra, the vagina and the anal canal pass through it.

 Short answer

22. 1. In general terms, describe the three important functions of the pelvic floor:

a. _____

b. _____

c. _____

2. Describe the influences the pelvic floor has during the childbirth process:

_____

_____

Muscle layers

The pelvic floor muscles are arranged into two layers, the superficial muscle layer (composed of five muscles) and the deep muscle layer (consists of four main pairs of muscles).

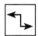 **Matching, colouring and labelling**

23. Figure 1.10 shows the superficial muscle layer of the pelvic floor. Using the key choices below, colour and label the superficial muscles and label the related structures and landmarks.

Colouring and labelling

Ischiocavernosa muscles
Transverse perineal muscle
Bulbocavernosus muscles
External anal sphincter
Membranous sphincter of urethra
Triangular ligament

Labelling

Coccyx
Clitoris
Urethral orifice
Ischial tuberosity
Vaginal orifice
Anus
Symphysis pubis

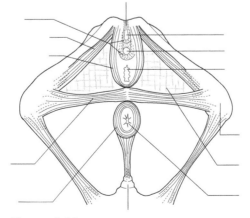

Figure 1.10

Completion

24. Using the information previously provided in Figure 1.10 now complete Table 1.5 by correctly inserting the key words from the extended list provided. Some words may be used more than once.

Ischial tuberosities	Anus	Anal sphincter	Urethra
Pubic bones	Vagina	Posteriorly	Perineum
Clitoris	Below	Ischial spines	Anteriorly
Pubic arch	Ischial tuberosities	Coccyx	Pubic bone
Above	Symphysis pubis		

Table 1.5

Superficial muscle	Describe the pathway of the muscle(s) and detail any structures of attachment involved
External anal sphincter	Encircles the _____ and is attached _____ by a few fibres to the _____.
Ischiocavernosus muscles	Passes from the _____ along the _____ to the corpora cavernosa.
Bulbocavernosus muscles	Passes from the perineum forwards around the _____ to the corpora cavernosa of the _____ just under the _____.
Transverse perineal muscles	Passes from the _____ to the centre of the _____.
Membranous sphincter of the urethra	Composed of muscle fibres passing _____ and _____ the _____ and attached to the _____ _____.

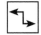 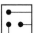 **Matching, colouring and labelling**

25. Figure 1.11 shows the deep muscle layer of the pelvic floor. Using the key choices below, match, colour and label the superficial muscles and label the related structures and landmarks.

Colouring and labelling

Pubococcygeus
Ischiococcygeus
Iliococcygeus

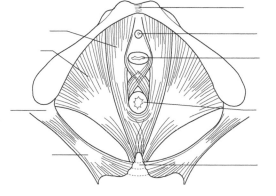

Colouring and labelling

Urethra
Vagina
Rectum

Labelling

Coccyx
Ischial spine
Symphysis pubis

Figure 1.11

Completion

26. Using the information previously provided in Figure 1.11 now complete Table 1.6 by ticking the statements most appropriate to the relevant muscle group(s). More than one column may be ticked.

Table 1.6

Statement	Deep muscles			
	Pubo-coccygeus	Pubo-rectalis	Ilio-coccygeus	Ischio-coccygeus
a. Passes around the rectum and continues to its insertion on the coccyx and lower sacrum				
b. It converges with the pubococcygeus where it inserts into the coccyx and lower sacrum				
c. It attaches to the coccyx, lower sacrum and median portion of the sacrotuberous ligament				
d. Originates from the fascial covering of the obturator internus muscle				
e. These muscle pairs become interlaced to the point of becoming inseparable				
f. It forms a horizontal sheet that spans the opening in the posterior region of the pelvis				
g. It forms a 'shelf' for pelvic organs to rest on				
h. Pass posteriorly encircling the rectum becoming part of the anorectal ring				
i. Originates from the ischial spine and adjacent sacroiliac fascia				

Miscelleneous questions about the pelvic floor

 True/false

27. Consider the following statements and choose if they are true or false by ticking the appropriate column. Provide a correct statement for those you have decided are false.

	Statement	True	False
a.	The pubococcygeus and the ischiococcygeus are collectively known as the levatores ani		
b.	Pelvic fascia is loose areolar tissue used like packaging material of spaces between and around muscle layers		
c.	The tissue that fills the triangular space between the bulbocavernosus and the iliocavernosus muscles is known as the triangular ligament		
d.	The perineal body, a pyramid of muscle and fibrous tissue, is located between the vaginal introitus and anus		
e.	The perineal body, a pyramid of muscle and fibrous tissue, measures 10 cm in each direction		
f.	The apex of the perineal body is formed from the fibres of the ischiocavernosus muscles		
g.	The base of the perineal body is formed from the transverse perineal muscles that meet in the perineum, together with the bulbocavernosus in front and the external anal sphincter behind		
h.	The external pudendal artery is the primary blood supply to the pelvis floor		
i.	Lymphatic drainage is through the common iliac nodes and the internal iliac nodes		
j.	The perineal body is stabilized by the rectovaginal septum (through its attachment to the cardinal and uterosacral ligaments) and also the lateral attachments of the lateral attachments of the perineal membrane to the ischiopubic rami		

2 The reproductive systems

The reproductive system in males and females differs in structure. The common function is primarily to ensure reproduction and the passing of the parents' genetic material to their children. Both systems produce gametes (sex cells) which fuse to form a potential human being. The female reproductive system has the additional role of protecting the developing fetus within the uterus, giving birth and nourishing the baby in the months after birth. This chapter will test your knowledge of the structures and some processes involved.

THE FEMALE REPRODUCTIVE SYSTEM

External structures of the female reproductive system

  Matching and labelling

1. The female reproductive system consists of the external genitalia and the internal reproductive organs. Figure 2.1 shows the external female genital organs. Label the structures by matching to the key options provided.

Anus
Clitoris
External urethral orifice
Frenum
Fourchette
Hymen
Labium minus
Labium majus

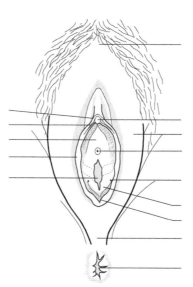

Mons veneris
Opening of Bartholin's duct
Perineum
Prepuce
Vagina
Vestibule

Figure 2.1

 Matching

2. The vulva is the collective term for the external genitalia. Each structure of the external genitalia has a unique description detailed in Table 2.1. Complete the following activity by matching the name of the structure from the list below to the correct description.

i. Mons pubis   ii. Vestibule   iii. Skene ducts

iv. Vaginal orifice   v. Hymen   vi. Bartholin's glands

vii. Labia majora   viii. Labia minora   ix. Prepuce

x. Urethral orifice

Table 2.1

	Description of structures of the vulva
a.	This area is enclosed by the labia minora in which the openings of the urethra and the vagina are situated.
b.	These secrete mucus which lubricates the vaginal opening.
c.	Anteriorly these two thin folds of skin divide to enclose the clitoris.
d.	This is a pad of fat lying over the symphysis pubis.
e.	These are two folds of fat and areolar tissue arising in the mons verenis and merging into the perineum behind.
f.	This is a retractable piece of skin surrounding and protecting the clitoris.
g.	This lies 2.5 cm posterior to the clitoris and immediately in front of the vaginal orifice.
h.	These are two small blind-ended tubules 0.5 cm long running within the urethral wall.
i.	This is thin membrane that tears during sexual intercourse or during the birth of the first baby.
j.	This structure occupies the posterior two-thirds of the vestibule.

Internal structures of the female reproductive system

  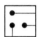 **Matching, colouring and labelling**

3. Figure 2.2 displays a coronal section through the pelvis. Label and colour the following structures and tissues by matching to the key options provided:

Label

Levator ani muscle
Ureter
Uterine tube
Vagina
Ovary
Uterus

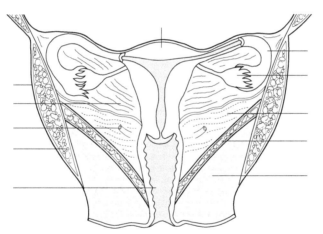

Label the other structures and tissues

Broad ligament
Pelvic fascia
Loose fat
Side wall of pelvis
Obturator internus muscle

Figure 2.2

4. Figure 2.3 presents a sagittal section of the female pelvis. Label and colour the following structures and tissues by matching to the key options provided:

Label

Urethra
Rectum
Uterus
Ureter
Perineal body
Bladder

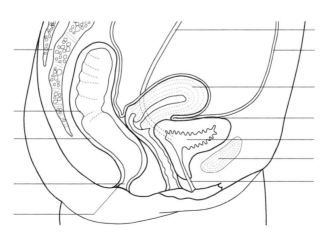

Label the other structures

Sacrum
Recto-uterine pouch of Douglas
Uterovesical pouch
Symphysis pubis
Anus
Peritoneum

Figure 2.3

5. Figure 2.4 shows the uterine tubes. Label and colour the following structures by matching to the key options provided:

Label

Ovary	Infundibulum with fimbriae	Fundus of uterus
Uterine tube	Ampulla	Vagina

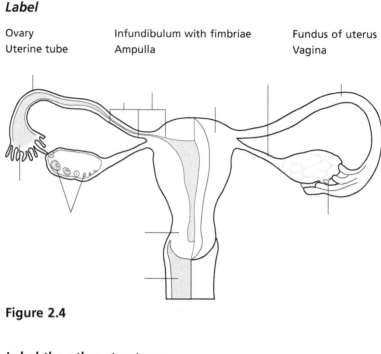

Figure 2.4

Label the other structures

Ovarian follicles	Cervix	Ovarian ligament
Isthmus	Interstitial portion	

6. Figure 2.5 shows the supports of the uterus at the level of the cervix. Label and colour the following structures by matching to the key options provided:

Rectum

Uterine cervix

Symphysis pubis

Transverse cervical ligament

Bladder

Uterosacral ligament

Pubocervical ligament

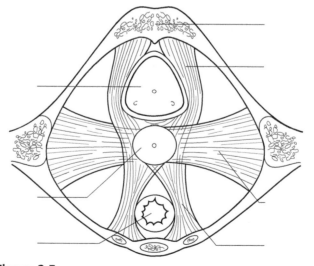

Figure 2.5

True/false

7. It is essential for practitioners to have detailed knowledge of structures within the female reproductive system. Consider the following statements in Table 2.2 and then decide which structure is referred to by ticking the appropriate column.

Table 2.2

	Statement	True	False
a.	The myometrium is thick in the upper part of the uterus and is sparser in the cervix and isthmus.		
b.	The body or corpus makes up one-third of the uterus.		
c.	The endometrium forms a lining of ciliated epithelium (mucous membrane) on a base of connective tissue.		
d.	The cervix stretches in labour due to the muscle fibres being embedded in collagen fibres.		
e.	The basal layer of the uterine layers alters due to the influence of hormones during the menstrual cycle.		
f.	When the woman stands upright, the vaginal canal points in an upward-backward direction and forms an angle of slightly more than 45° with the uterus.		
g.	The uterovesical pouch lies between the bladder and uterus and is formed by the perimetrium draping over the anterior surface of the uterus reflecting onto the bladder.		
h.	The perimetrium is the innermost layer of the uterus.		
i.	Lymphatic drainage of the uterus provides an effective defence against uterine infection.		
j.	The fibres of the myometrium interlace to surround the blood vessels that pass to and from the endometrium.		
k.	The ovaries are attached to the back of the broad ligament.		
l.	Bartholin's glands lie in the anterior part of the labia majora.		
m.	The vaginal walls are thrown into small folds known as rugae.		
n.	The ovary is supported from above by the ovarian ligament medially and the infundibulopelvic ligament laterally.		
o.	After childbirth the internal os becomes a transverse slit.		
p.	The ovary is composed of a cortex and medulla.		
q.	During pregnancy the isthmus of the uterus enlarges to form the lower uterine segment.		

The uterus and uterine tubes

 Completion

8. The paragraph below describes aspects of the uterus. Cross out the incorrect options so that the paragraph reads correctly:

The uterus is a hollow **pear/oval**-shaped **muscular/visceral** organ located in the **true/false** pelvis between the **bladder/kidney** and the **vagina/rectum**. The position of the uterus within the **true/false** pelvis is one of **ante/retro**-version and **ante/retro**-flexion. **Ante/retro**-version means that the uterus leans forward and **ante/retro**-flexion means that it bends forwards upon itself. When the woman is standing, the uterus is in an almost **horizontal/lateral** position with the **cervix/fundus** resting on the bladder.

 Multiple choice questions (MCQs)

9. The uterine tubes are also known as:

   a. Oviducts

   b. Fallopian tubes

   c. Salpinges

   d. All of the above

10. The transverse cervical ligaments are sometimes known as:

   a.   Cardinal ligaments

   b.   Broad ligaments

   c.   Mackenrodt's ligaments

   d.   a and c

   e.   None of the above

11. The ampulla of the uterine tube is:

   a.   The wider portion and is 5 cm long

   b.   The narrow portion and is 2 cm long

   c.   The funnel-shaped portion and is 5 cm long

   d.   None of the above

Short answers

12. Provide the following numerical values:

   a.   Measurements of the vagina:

      i.   Diameter _____ cm

      ii. Length of posterior wall _____ cm

      iii. Length of anterior wall _____ cm

   b.   Measurements of the non-pregnant uterus:

      i.   Length _____ cm

      ii. Width _____ cm

      iii. Depth_____ cm

      iv. Thickness of each wall_____ cm

   c.   Measurement of each uterine tube: length _____ cm

   d.   What is the pH value of vaginal fluid? pH _____

13. Describe how the pH value of the vaginal fluid is created: _____

   _____

   _____

14. The labia minora are also known as: _____

15. The labia majora are also known as: _____

16. The upper end of the vagina is known as the: _____

17. Name the three layers of the vagina:

a.   _____

b.   _____

c.   _____

18. Name the four portions of the uterine tube:

a.   _____   b.   _____

c.   _____   d.   _____

Completion

19. Complete the following paragraph by inserting the missing word(s) from the list provided so that the paragraph reads correctly.

ciliated cubical epithelium	circular
glycogen	goblet cells
longitudinal	oocyte
peristaltic movement	plicae
slow down	smooth muscle

The lining of the uterine tubes is mucous membrane of _____ that is thrown

into folds known as _____. These folds _____ the ovum on its way to

the uterus. There are _____ within the lining that produce a secretion containing

_____ to nourish the _____. The muscle coat consists of two

layers, an inner _____ layer and an outer _____ layer. Both

layers are composed of _____ which produce _____

of the tube.

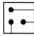 **Matching and labelling**

20. Figure 2.6 shows a cross section of a uterine tube and ovary. Label the diagram by matching to only nine of the anatomical structures listed below:

Ovary
Circular muscle
Longitudinal muscle
Oblique muscle
Ciliated cubical epithelium
Ovarian blood vessels

Smooth muscle
Peritoneum (perisalpinx)
Mesovarium
Lumen of tube
Mucous membrane
Myometrium

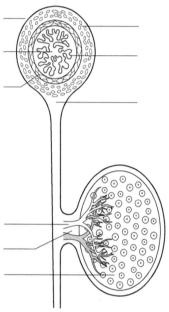

Figure 2.6

THE MALE REPRODUCTIVE SYSTEM

The male reproductive organs

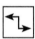 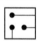 **Matching, colouring and labelling**

21. Figure 2.7 shows the male reproductive organs. Some organs are partly visible and others are partly hidden within the body.

Label and/or colour the following structures

Urethra
Testis
Urinary bladder
Scrotum
Prostrate gland

Label these other structures

Ejaculatory duct
Seminal vesicle
Corpus cavernosum
Penis
Spermatic cord and deferent duct
Prepuce
Glans penis
Deferent duct
Bulbourethral gland
Corpus spongiosum
Epididymis

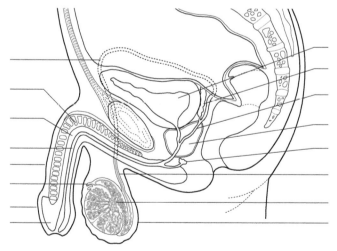

Figure 2.7

True/false

22. Consider the following statements in Table 2.3 and choose if they are true or false by ticking the appropriate column.

Table 2.3

	Statement	True	False
a.	The prostate is an endocrine gland of the male reproductive system.		
b.	The scrotum forms a pouch in which the testes are suspended outside the body keeping them at a temperature lower than the rest of the body.		
c.	The control of the male gonads is cyclical.		
d.	Mature sperm are stored in the epididymis and the deferent duct until ejaculation.		
e.	Seminal fluid contains about 1 million sperm/mL of which 30% are likely to be abnormal.		
f.	The testes are the body's main source of the male hormone testosterone.		
g.	Spermatogenesis takes place in the seminiferous tubules.		
h.	Normal spermatozoon move at a speed of 2–3 mm/min.		
i.	Testes are components of both the reproductive system and the endocrine system.		

 Multiple choice questions (MCQs)

23. Spermatogenesis takes place under the influence of:

   a. Follicle stimulating hormone (FSH) only

   b. Testosterone only

   c. Thyroxine

   d. Testosterone and follicle stimulating hormone (FSH)

24. The ideal temperature for the production of viable sperm is:

   a. 34.4°C   b. 35.5 °C   c. 36.7 °C   d. 33.6 °C

The female urinary tract

The urinary system is an important excretory system that plays a vital role in maintaining homeostasis (together with other body systems) of water and electrolyte concentrations in the body. The urinary tract begins with the kidneys, and continues as a passage for urine in the ureters, the bladder and the urethra. This chapter will help you to understand how this occurs.

The structure and functions of the kidney

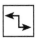   **Matching, colouring and labelling**

1. The kidneys are a pair of bean-shaped excretory glands. Figure 3.1 shows the longitudinal section of the kidney. Label and colour the following structures and label the other structures and tissues by matching to options provided:

Label and colour

Pelvis of kidney
Renal vein
Renal artery
Ureter

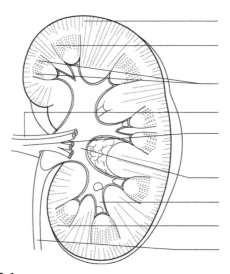

Label

Cortex
Medulla
Medullary rays
Calyx
Column of Bertini

Figure 3.1

 Completion

2. The functions of the kidney can be summarized into the categories of elimination, regulation and secretion. Complete Table 3.1 by listing six broad functions of the kidneys.

Table 3.1

	Six broad functions of the kidneys
i.	Elimination of
ii.	Elimination of
iii.	Regulation of
iv.	Regulation of
v.	Regulation of
vi.	Secretion of

The basic functional unit of the kidney

 Completion

3. The paragraphs below relate to the nephron which is the basic functional unit of the kidney. Each nephron starts as a knot of capillaries called a glomerulus. Surrounding the glomerulus is a cup known as the glomerular capsule. Together the glomerulus and capsule are known as the glomerular body. Cross out the incorrect options so that the paragraphs read correctly:

The glomerulus is fed by a branch of the renal artery, the **efferent/afferent** arteriole, and the blood is collected into the **efferent/afferent** arteriole. The pressure within the glomerulus is **raised/lowered** because the **efferent/afferent** arteriole has a wider bore than the **efferent/afferent** arteriole. This factor forces the filtrate **into/out of** the capillaries **out of/into** the capsule. At this stage any substance with a **small/large** molecular size will be filtered out.

The cup of the capsule is first attached to a tubule that has three distinct regions before joining the straight collecting duct receiving urine. The first region of the tubule is the twisting **proximal convoluted tubule/distal convoluted tubule/loop of Henle**, the middle region is the straight **proximal convoluted tubule/distal convoluted tubule/loop of Henle**, and the third region before joining the collecting duct is the twisting **proximal convoluted tubule/distal convoluted tubule/loop of Henle**.

   Matching, colouring and labelling

4. Figure 3.2 shows a glomerular body. Label the structures from the list provided.

Afferent arteriole
Distal convoluted tubule
Efferent arteriole
Glomerulus
Glomerular capsule
Granular juxtaglomerular cells
Macula dorsa
Proximal convoluted tubule

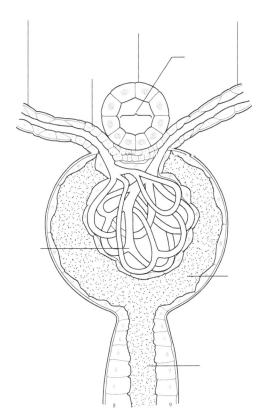

Figure 3.2

5. Figure 3.3 shows a nephron. Label, colour and match the structures as detailed below:

Colour and label

Afferent arteriole
Efferent arteriole
Branch of renal artery
Branch of renal vein

Label

Glomerular bodies
Distal convoluted tubule
Proximal convoluted tubule
Medulla
Cortex
Straight collecting tubule
Loop of Henle
Capillary

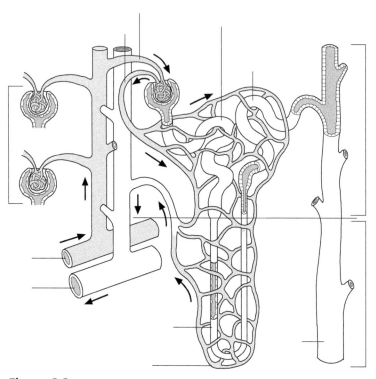

Figure 3.3

? Multiple choice questions (MCQs)

6. The adult kidneys are about:

    a. 10 cm long, 6.5 cm wide, 3 cm thick and weigh 120 g

    b. 5 cm long, 10 cm wide, 6 cm thick and weigh 70 g

    c. 15 cm long, 10 cm wide, 10 cm thick and weigh 170 g

    d. 6 cm long, 3 cm wide, 2 cm thick and weigh 50 g

7. In the healthy adult kidney there are:

    a. 500 000 nephrons

    b. 1 million nephrons

    c. 5 million nephrons

    d. 10 million nephrons

8. The main structures (renal artery, renal vein, nerves and lymphatics) enter and leave the kidney at the:

    a. Medulla   b. Capsule   c. Hilum   d. Cortex

9. In the nephron filtration takes place in the:

    a. Glomerulus

    b. Distal convoluted tubule

    c. Proximal convoluted tubule

    d. Loop of Henle

10. Which options contain only normal constituents of filtrate?

a. Water, salts and glucose

b. Water, blood components and salts

c. Blood corpuscles, platelets and plasma proteins

d. Blood corpuscles, salts and glucose

11. Of the vast amount of fluid that passes out in the filtrate daily, how much is reabsorbed?

a. Less than 1%

b. About 10%

c. 50%

d. 99%

12. Antidiuretic hormone (ADH) is produced by the:

a. Anterior pituitary gland

b. Posterior pituitary gland

c. Kidney

d. Cortex of the suprarenal gland

13. Aldosterone is produced in the:

a. Anterior pituitary gland

b. Posterior pituitary gland

c. Kidney

d. Cortex of the suprarenal gland

14. The reabsorption of sodium is primarily controlled by:

a. Antidiuretic hormone

b. Aldosterone

c. Calcitonin

d. Adrenaline

The bladder, ureters and ligaments

  Matching and labelling

15. Figure 3.4 shows a section through the bladder. Label the structures from the list of options provided.

Bell's muscle
Internal urethral orifice
Interureteric bar
Opening of the ureter
Rugae
Trigone
Ureter
Urethra

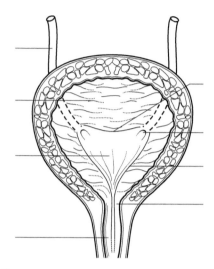

Figure 3.4

 Completion

16. Complete the following activity by inserting the missing word(s) and numerical values from the extended list provided so that it reads correctly:

anterior	front	muscle	posterior	vagina
apex	globular	outer	pyramidal	lining
back	hilum	peristalsis	trigone	round
3	25	30	50	300
600	1000	2000		

The ureters are composed of three layers: a _____, a _____ layer and an _____

coat. At the upper end of the urinary tract, the ureter is continuous with the renal _____ of the kidney

and runs to the _____ wall of the bladder. Each tube is about _____ mm in diameter and

between ____ and ____ cm in length. The ureters transport urine to the bladder by _____.

The shape of the bladder is described as being _____ when empty and becomes more

_____ in shape as it becomes filled with urine. The base of the bladder is termed the

_____. It is situated at the _____ of the bladder and rests against the _____. The

capacity of the bladder is around _____ ml.

17. Complete the following Table 3.2 by providing correct missing information about the five ligaments (two pairs and one single) attached to the bladder.

Table 3.2

	Name of ligament(s)	Extend(s) from:	To:
a.		bladder neck anteriorly	
b.			side walls of the pelvis
c.		apex of bladder	

True/false

18. Consider the following statements in Table 3.3 and indicate if they are true or false by ticking the appropriate column.

Table 3.3

	Statement	True	False
a.	The kidneys only have an exocrine function.		
b.	Renin and erythropoietin are hormones secreted by the kidney.		
c.	Erythropoietin stimulates the production of red blood cells.		
d.	The specific gravity of urine is 1.010–1.030.		
e.	Urine is acidic.		
f.	Urine consists of 90% water, 5% urea and 5% other solutes.		
g.	The anterior part of the bladder lies close to the symphysis pubis and is termed the apex.		
h.	The right kidney is longer and more slender than the left kidney.		
i.	A low bacterial count of less than 100 000/ml is not significant to confirm a urinary tract infection.		
j.	The absence of ADH causes segments of the kidney's tubule system to become more permeable to water.		
k.	Certain substances such as creatinine and toxins are added directly to urine in the ascending arm of the loop of Henle.		
l.	The hormone renin is produced in the afferent arteriole and is secreted in response to a reduced blood supply and in response to low sodium levels.		
m.	During pregnancy, stasis of urine can result due to the relaxation influence progesterone has on the walls of the ureters.		
n.	In the days following birth, there is a rapid and sustained loss of sodium and a major dieresis occurs.		
o.	Glomerular filtration is reduced during pregnancy to compensate for the additional maternal and fetal metabolism.		
p.	The right kidney is located slightly lower than the left kidney.		
q.	Renal agenesis refers to the congenital absence of one or two kidneys.		

4 Hormonal cycles: fertilization and early development

The female hormonal cycles commence at puberty and are monthly physiological changes that take place in the ovaries and the uterus, regulated by hormones produced by the hypothalamus, pituitary gland and ovaries. These cycles occur simultaneously and together they are known as the female reproductive cycle. This chapter will help you to understand how this occurs and the processes involved.

Ovarian cycle

 Completion

1. The following paragraphs below relate to the three phases of the ovarian cycle which are all under the control of hormones. Cross out the incorrect options so that the paragraphs read correctly.

Phase One

In the **follicular/luteal** phase low levels of ovarian hormones stimulate the **ovaries/hypothalamus** to produce **gonadotrophin releasing hormone (GnRH)/ovarian hormones**. This hormone causes the production of **oestrogen/follicle stimulating hormone (FSH)** and **luteinizing hormone (LH)/progesterone** by the **anterior/posterior** pituitary gland. Under the influence of this hormone, the Graafian follicle secretes **oestrogen/progesterone** and as a result there is a surge in **LH/FSH**. When hormone levels reach a certain peak, the secretion of **LH/FSH** is inhibited. Eventually the largest and most dominant follicle secretes inhibin, which further suppresses **FSH/LH**, and this follicle prevails and becomes competent to ovulate. The time from growth and maturity of the Graafian follicles to ovulation is normally around **one/two** week(s), i.e. day **5–14/10–21** of a 28-day cycle of events.

Phase Two

Ovulation is stimulated by a sudden **surge/reduction** in **LH/progesterone** which matures the **oocyte/corpus luteum**. This occurs around day **2–4/12–13** of a 28-day cycle and lasts for **48 hours/72 hours**.

Phase Three

In the final **follicular/luteal** phase, the **corpus luteum/corpus albicans** is formed by **proliferation/recession** of the residual ruptured follicle. This is a **yellow/white** irregular structure producing **oestrogen/LH** and **progesterone/FSH** for approximately **2/4** weeks. This develops the **endometrium/myometrium** which awaits the fertilized oocyte. The **corpus luteum/corpus albicans** continues its role until the **placenta/endometrium** is developed adequately to take over. If fertilization does not occur then the **corpus luteum/corpus albicans** degenerates and becomes the **corpus luteum/corpus albicans**. There is a decrease in **oestrogen and progesterone/FSH/LH hormones** and inhibin levels. These low hormone levels stimulate the **pituitary gland/hypothalamus** to produce **GnRH/FSH**. Rising levels of these hormones stimulate the **anterior/posterior** pituitary gland to produce **FSH/LH** and the cycle begins again.

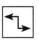 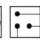 **Matching, colouring and labelling**

2. Figure 4.1 presents the cycle of a Graafian follicle in the ovary. Label Figure 4.1 from the words listed above and below the Figure:

| Developing corpus luteum | Fully developed corpus luteum | Ovarian ligament | Ovulation-released oocyte | Follicle reaching maturity |

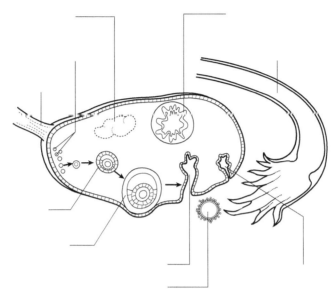

Figure 4.1

| Uterine tube | Ruptured follicle | Large pre-ovulatory follicle | Developing follicles | Corpus albicans |

3. Figure 4.2 shows a ripe Graafian follicle. Label Figure 4.2 from the options below:

Granulosa cells
Oocyte
Zona pellucida
Theca
External limiting membrane
Follicular fluid
Corona radiata
Stroma of ovary
Discus proligerus
Perivitelline space

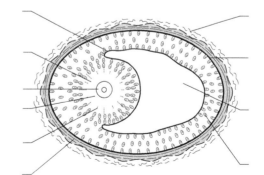

Figure 4.2

Female reproductive cycle and fertilization

  ## Colouring and labelling

4. Figure 4.3 details the female reproductive cycle during the menstrual cycle and early pregnancy. Carefully consider each section of this figure. Label the processes/structures involved from the list provided.

1. Blastocyst 2. Embedded 'trophoblast' 3. Fertilization 4. Morula 5. Oocyte 6. Segmentation

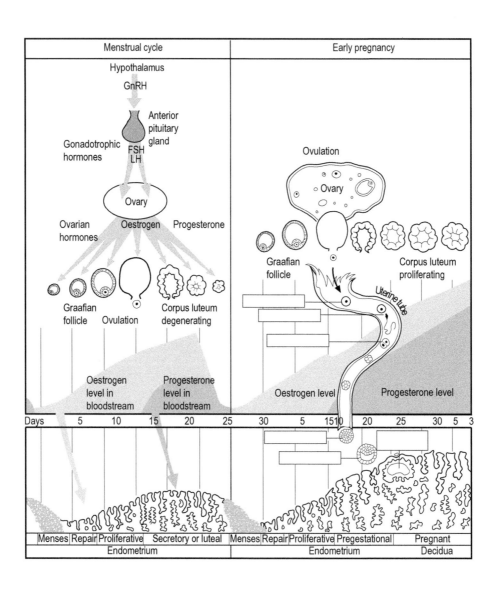

Figure 4.3

Completion

5. The menstrual cycle or endometrial cycle refers to the physiological changes that occur in the uterus in preparation to receive the fertilized oocyte. The cycle consists of three phases: menstrual, proliferative and secretory phases. Consider the following statements in Table 4.1 and tick the appropriate phase the statement applies to.

Table 4.1

Descriptive statement	Menstrual phase	Proliferative phase	Secretory phase
a. It is simultaneous with ovulation.			
b. Physiologically this is the terminal phase of the reproductive cycle.			
c. It is simultaneous with the beginning of the follicular phase of the ovarian cycle.			
d. At the end of this phase the endometrium consists of three layers.			
e. The fertilized oocyte implants itself within the endometrium.			
f. The spiral arteries of the endometrium go into spasm.			
g. The functional layer of the endometrium thickens to approximately 3.5 mm thick.			
h. It follows the proliferative phase.			
i. The functional layer, which contains tubular glands, is approximately 2.5 mm thick.			
j. It is under the influence of progesterone and oestrogen secreted by the corpus luteum.			
k. Eumenorrhoea occurs.			
l. There is the formation of a new layer of endometrium.			
m. The blood supply to the area is increased			
n. There is necrosis of the endometrium.			
o. It is under the control of oestradiol and other oestrogens secreted by the Graafian follicle.			
p. Some women experience dysmenorrhoea.			
q. The regenerative phase occurs.			
r. A layer of cuboidal ciliated epithelium covers the functional layer.			
s. Glands produce nutritive secretions.			

Early development following fertilization

  Matching, colouring and labelling

6. Figure 4.4 depicts the development of the blastocyst at 13 days (smaller diagram) and then again at 18 days. In the smaller diagram (blastocyst 13 days) label and colour the following structures:

Label and colour

Yolk sac
Amniotic sac
Syncytiotrophoblast

Label

Ectoderm
Mesoderm
Embryonic plate
Endoderm
Cytotrophoblast

Label and colour

Amniotic sac
Embryo
Yolk sac
Chorion

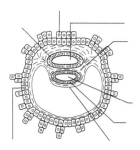

Blastocyst 13 days

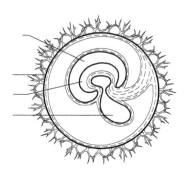

Blastocyst 18 days

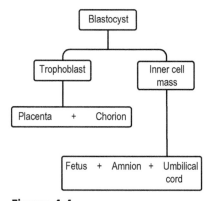

Figure 4.4

Completion

7. The following paragraph relates to fertilization. Cross out the incorrect word(s) so that the paragraph reads correctly.

Once inside the uterine tubes the sperm undergo changes to the plasma membrane resulting in the removal of the glycoprotein coat. The **acrosomal/cortical** layer of the sperm becomes reactive with the release of the enzyme **hyaluronidase/hydrogenase** and this is known as the **acrosome/cortical** reaction. This disperses the outermost layer of the oocyte called **corona radiata/zona pellucida** allowing access to the **corona radiata/zona pellucida.** The first sperm that reaches the **zona pellucida/cortical layer** penetrates it with the aid of several enzymes. Upon penetration **acrosomal/cortical** reaction occurs which makes the **zona pellucida/cortical layer** impermeable to other sperm. The **plasma membranes/nuclei** of the oocyte and sperm fuse. The oocyte at this stage completes its **first/second** meiotic division and becomes **immature/mature.**

 Short answers

8. Explain the following terms related to the process of fertilization:

a. Haploid: _____

_____

b. Diploid: _____

_____

c. Zygote: _____

_____

Development of the zygote

✎ Completion

9. The following section relates to the development of the zygote. Complete the missing words/phrases from the list provided. Note that some words may be used more than once.

Decidua	Cleavage	Blastocyst	Morula
Blastomeres	Trophoblast	Inner cell mass	Uterus
Compaction	Cavitation	Blastocele	Mitotic
Outer cell mass	Placenta	Amnion	Embryo
Embryoblast	Umbilical cord		

During the journey along the uterine tube the zygote undergoes _____ cellular replication and

division referred to as _____ resulting in smaller cells known as _____. The zygote

divides into two cells at day 1, four at day 2, eight by 2.5 days and sixteen by 3 days, now known as the

_____. The cells bind together in a process known as _____. Next

_____ occurs whereby the outermost cells secrete fluid into the _____ and

a fluid filled cavity or _____ appears in the _____. This results in the formation

of the _____ that enters the _____ around day 3–5. The _____ possesses

an _____ or _____ and an _____ or

_____. Implantation of the _____ layer occurs into the endometrium, and

this is now known as the_____. The _____ or _____ becomes

the _____ and chorion while the _____ or _____ becomes the

_____, _____ and umbilical cord.

10. During the development of the zygote the epiblast cells give rise to the cells of the embryo. There are three layers which form particular parts of the embryo. Complete the following Table 4.2 and give examples of the parts of the embryo developed from each layer.

Table 4.2

Layer	Parts of the embryo developed
a. Ectoderm	This is the start of tissue that
b. Mesoderm	This forms
c. Endoderm	This forms

True/false

11. Consider the following statements in Table 4.3 and indicate if they are true or false by ticking the appropriate column.

Table 4.3

	Statement	True	False
a.	Under the influence of oestrogen the cervix secretes a flow of alkaline mucus that attracts the spermatozoa.		
b.	Human fertilization, known as conception, is the fusion of the sperm with the secondary oocyte to form the zygote.		
c.	Blastulation occurs around day 4 and refers to the process involved in the development of the morula to the blastocyst.		
d.	The syncytiotrophoblast layer of the trophoblast cells or syncitium invade the decidua by forming villi.		
e.	The oocyte moves along the uterine tube by the action of cilia and peristalsis.		
f.	Mittleschmerz is the term that refers to the varying degrees of abdominal pain experienced by women during ovulation.		
g.	Implantation is usually in the upper anterior wall of the uterus.		
h.	Once inside the uterine tubes the sperm undergo a process known as decapacitation.		
i.	The syncytiotrophoblast cells produce human gonadotrophin (hCG) hormone.		
j.	In the healthy fertile male at intercourse approximately 3 million sperm are deposited in the posterior fornix of the vagina.		
k.	Hypoblast layer of the embryoblast give rise to extra-amniotic structures only such as the yolk sac.		
l.	Many of the sperm are destroyed by the alkaline medium in the vagina.		
m.	Lacunae are spaces in the decidua that fill up with maternal blood.		
n.	The pre-embryonic period is crucial in terms of initiation and maintenance of pregnancy and early embryonic development.		
o.	After birth, the only remains of the yolk sac is the vitelline duct at the base of the umbilical cord.		

? Multiple choice questions (MCQs)

12. The process of human fertilization normally takes approximately:

    a. 1 hour

    b. 24 hours

    c. 48 hours

    d. 4 hours

13. Human fertilization normally occurs in the:

    a. Fimbria of the uterine tube

    b. Fundus of the uterus

    c. Ampulla of the uterine tube

    d. Isthmus of the uterine tube

14. The embryoblast cells:

    a. Differentiate into epiblasts (closest to the trophoblast)

    b. Differentiate into hypoblasts (closest to the blastocyst cavity)

    c. Give rise to cells of the embryo

    d. All of the above

15. Following fertilization, the first appearance of the primitive streak is around:

    a. 2 days   b. 10 days   c. 15 days   d. 20 days

The fully developed placenta is a vital and complex organ which serves as the interface between the mother and the developing fetus. The survival of the fetus depends upon the integrity and efficiency of the placenta, membranes and umbilical cord. This chapter will help you to understand the development, function and processes involved.

Early development of the placenta

 Labelling

1. Figure 5.1 shows the chorionic villi. Match and label the structures and tissues from the list provided.

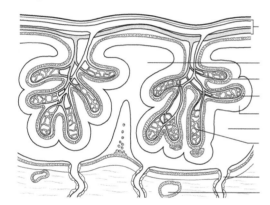

Decidual gland
Cytotrophoblast
Fetal capillary
Syncytiotrophoblast
Intervillous spaces (×2)
Fetal vessels leading from and to umbilical vessels
Mesoderm
Maternal vessel

Figure 5.1

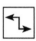 **Matching, colouring and labelling**

2. Figure 5.2 shows the blood flow around the chorionic villi. Colour and label the structures and tissues from the options provided.

Label and colour

Umbilical vein
Umbilical artery
Maternal vein
Decidua

Label

Main villus
Septum
Maternal spiral artery
Uterine muscle

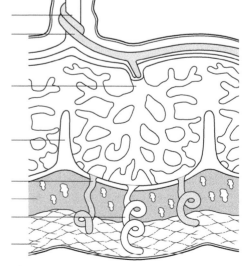

Figure 5.2

Completion

3. Flow diagram 5.1 relates to the early development of the placenta. Complete the missing words by matching the correct terminology from the list provided below. A small number of words are used more than once.

blastocyst	chorionic villi	decidua parietalis
blood spaces	cytokines	placenta
chorion frondosum	decidua	protease inhibitors
chorion laeve	decidua basilis	trophoblasts
chorionic membrane	decidua capsularis	sinuses

Flow diagram 5.1: Early development of the placenta

a. By 10 days, the _____ is completely buried in the decidua. The _____ have a potent invasive capacity. The decidua secretes _____ and _____ that moderate this invasion.

↓

b. _____ form from the proliferation of projections from the trophoblastic layer from about 3 weeks after fertilization. This becomes more profuse in the _____ where there is a rich blood supply. This is known as the _____ which develops into the _____.

↓

c. The portion of deciduas surrounding the _____ where it projects into the uterine cavity is known as the _____. The villi under this area degenerates forming _____ _____ from where the _____ originates. The remaining decidua is known as the _____.

↓

d. As the uterus is filled with the enlarging fetus the _____ thins and disappears and the chorion meets the _____ on the opposite wall of the uterus.

↓

e. The villi penetrate the _____ and erode the walls of maternal blood vessels opening them up to form a lake of maternal blood in which they float. The opened blood vessels are known as _____ and the area surrounding the villi are called _____.

The mature placenta

 Completion

4. The placenta performs a variety of functions for the developing fetus. List six key functions:

_____   _____

_____   _____

_____   _____

5. This question relates to placental circulation. Complete the paragraphs below by choosing the appropriate words to read correctly:

Maternal blood is discharged into the intervillous space by **25–50/80–100** spiral arteries. Blood flows **slowly/quickly** around the villi, eventually returning to the endometrial **veins/arteries** and the maternal circulation. There are about **75 ml/150 ml** of maternal blood in the intervillous spaces, which is exchanged **3 or 4/7 or 8** times per minute.

Fetal blood, **high/low** in oxygen, is pumped by the fetal heart towards the placenta along the umbilical **vein/arteries** and transported along their branches to the capillaries of the chorionic villi where exchange of nutrients takes place between mother and fetus. Having yielded up **oxygen/carbon dioxide** and waste products and absorbed **carbon dioxide/oxygen** and nutrients the blood is returned to the fetus via the umbilical **arteries/vein.**

True/false

6. Consider the following statements in Table 5.1 and indicate if they are true or false by ticking the appropriate column.

Table 5.1

	Statement	True	False
a.	Between 12 and 20 weeks' gestation the placenta weighs less than the fetus.		
b.	Carbon dioxide is the main substance excreted from the placenta.		
c.	The cytotrophoblast cells and the syncytiotrophoblast gradually degenerate as some of the fetal organs such as the liver develop.		
d.	The placenta can also store iron and fat-soluble vitamins.		
e.	Oxygen from the maternal haemoglobin does not pass directly into the fetal blood by simple diffusion.		
f.	Fat soluble vitamins (A, C, D, and E) cross the placenta.		
g.	Carbon dioxide passes into maternal blood by simple diffusion.		
h.	Nutrients are actively transferred from maternal to fetal blood through the walls of the villi.		
i.	The placenta provides only a limited barrier to infection.		
j.	Amino acids are found at higher levels in the fetal blood than in maternal blood.		

Short answers

7. Name the two types of villi:

_____ villi and _____ villi.

8. Name the one bacteria that can cross the placenta: _____

9. Name two viruses that can cross the placenta:

_____   _____

10. Name the four key hormones produced by the placenta:

_____   _____

_____   _____

Matching

11. Complete the following statements about nutritional function of the mature placenta in Table 5.2 by choosing the correct term from the list provided.

i. Blood formation   ii. Glycogen   iii. Body building

iv. Bones and teeth   v. Energy and growth   vi. Bilirubin

Table 5.2

a. Amino acids are required for
b. Calcium and phosphorus are required for
c. Glucose is required for
d. The placenta stores glucose in the form of
e. The placenta excretes carbon dioxide and also excretes
f. Iron is required for

Placental membranes

Completion

12. The following words/phrases relate to either the amnion or chorion membrane. Consider and then match them to the appropriate membrane.

a. Outer membrane   b. Inner membrane   c. Smooth   d. Tough

e. Thick   f. Translucent   g. Inner cell mass   h. Friable

i. Derived from the trophoblast   j. Opaque   k. Lines the surface of the placenta   l. Continues with the outer surface of the umbilical cord

i.   Chorion: _____

_____

_____

ii.   Amnion: _____

_____

_____

Amniotic fluid

✎ Short answers

13. List the main functions of amniotic fluid a) during pregnancy b) in labour (intact):

   a. During pregnancy

_____

_____

_____

_____

   b. In labour (intact)

_____

_____

_____

The structure of the mature placenta

It is important that midwives have detailed knowledge of the structure of the placenta at term.

✎ Completion

14. Complete the approximate measurements of the placenta:

   a. Diameter: _____ cm.

   b. Thickness at the centre: _____cm.

   c. The weight is about _____ th of the baby's weight.

Matching

15. Consider the following statements in Table 5.3 about the placental surfaces. Match the statements to the relevant surface by ticking the appropriate column.

Table 5.3

Statements	Maternal surface	Fetal surface
a. It has a shiny appearance.		
b. Branches of the umbilical vein and arteries are visible.		
c. It is arranged into cotyledons (lobes).		
d. It is covered by amnion.		
e. It is dark red in colour.		
f. The amnion can be peeled off the surface of the chorion to the umbilical cord.		
g. Sulci separate cotyledons (lobes).		
h. Umbilical cord insertion is located.		
i. Decidua dips down into sulci to form septa.		
j. Sometimes lime salts may be present.		

Umbilical cord

 Completion

16. Complete the following questions and statements about the umbilical cord:

   a. Detail the number and name of the blood vessels contained in the umbilical cord:

   i. No of vessels: _____

   ii. Names of vessels: _____

   b. What substance encloses and protects the umbilical blood vessels: _____

   c. The diameter of the cord is approximately: i. _____ cm and the length of the cord is ii. ____–____ cm.

   d. Describe the disadvantages of a very long cord:

   _____

   _____

Anatomical variations of placenta and cord

 Short answers

17. The following two figures relate to anatomical variations of the placenta and cord. Name and describe the type of variation including how it is formed (if appropriate) and identify associated risks:

   a. Figure 5.3

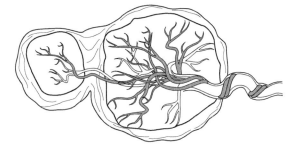

Figure 5.3

Name and describe: _____

_____

_____

_____

Associated risk factors: _____

_____

_____

b. Figure 5.4

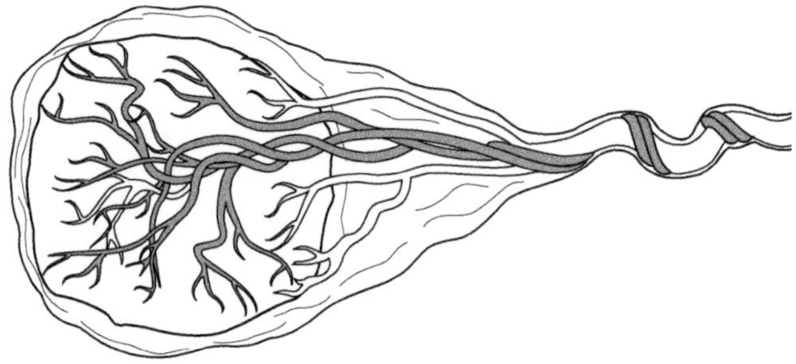

Figure 5.4

Name and describe: _____

_____

_____

_____

Associated risk factors: _____

_____

_____

? Multiple choice questions (MCQs)

18. The placenta is completely formed and functioning in:

   a. 8 weeks after fertilization

   b. 10 weeks after fertilization

   c. 12 weeks after fertilization

   d. 14 weeks after fertilization

19. Antibodies in the form of immunoglobulin G (IgG) transferred to the placenta offer the baby passive immunity for the first:

    a. 1 month

    b. 2 months

    c. 3 months

    d. 6 months

20. Maternal and fetal blood is separated by:

    a. Two layers of tissues

    b. Three layers of tissues

    c. Four layers of tissues

    d. Six layers of tissues

21. Amniotic fluid is thought to be:

    a. Exuded from maternal vessels in the deciduas

    b. Exuded from fetal vessels in the placenta

    c. Secreted by the amnion

    d. All of the above

22. The water in amniotic fluid is exchanged approximately:

    a. Hourly

    b. Three-hourly

    c. Six-hourly

    d. Daily

23. The volume of amniotic fluid is greatest at approximately:

    a. 36 weeks' gestation

    b. 38 weeks' gestation

    c. 40 weeks' gestation

    d. None of the above

6 The fetus

This chapter focuses on fetal growth and development, the fetal circulation and fetal skull. Knowledge of fetal development is essential to fully understand the situation for babies born both preterm and term. This chapter will help you to assess your knowledge in these areas.

FETAL DEVELOPMENT

Development of the embryo

 Completion

1. Embryological development is complex and occurs from week 2 to 8 after fertilization followed by fetal development until the birth of the baby. The following statements in Table 6.1 relate to embryological or fetal development up to 20 weeks' gestation. Complete the following table by ticking the appropriate gestational age range for each statement.

Table 6.1

Development of embryological and fetal development	Weeks of gestation				
	0–4	4–8	8–12	12–16	16–20
a. Gender distinguishable					
b. Limb buds form					
c. Primitive streak appears					
d. **Rapid** weight gain					
e. 'Quickening' – mother feels fetal movements					
f. Meconium present in gut					
g. Swallowing begins					
h. Urine passed					
i. Fetal heart heard on auscultation					
j. Vernix caseosa appears					
k. Nasal septum and palate fuse					
l. Lanugo appears					
m. Early movements					

Development of the fetus

2. The following statements in Table 6.2 relate to fetal development from 20 weeks' gestation until the birth of the baby. Consider the statements and complete the following table by ticking the appropriate gestational age range for each statement.

Table 6.2

Development of fetal development	Weeks of gestation				
	20–24	24–28	28–32	32–36	36–birth
a. Testes descend into scrotum					
b. Head hair lengthens					
c. Responds to sound					
d. Eyelids open					
e. Skin red and wrinkled					
f. Respiratory movements					
g. Begins to store fat and iron					
h. Plantar creases visible					
i. Skull formed but soft and pliable					
j. Lanugo disappears from body					
k. Increased fat makes body more rounded					
l. Weight gain 25 g/day					

The placenta is the source of oxygenation, nutrition and excretion of waste products of metabolism for the fetus. In addition there are several temporary structures that enable the fetal circulation to occur. Sound knowledge of the structures and processes involved in the fetal circulation and adaptation to extrauterine life is essential.

Fetal circulation

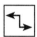   **Matching, colouring and labelling**

3. Figure 6.1 presents a diagram of the fetal circulation. Match, colour and label the structures as listed below.

Label and colour

Superior vena cava
Inferior vena cava
Umbilical vein
Aorta
Pulmonary artery
Pulmonary veins

Label

Ductus arteriosus
Ductus venosus
Foramen ovale
Left lung
Renal vein
Umbilicus
Renal artery
Hypogastric arteries
Liver
Portal vein
Umbilicus arteries
Right lung

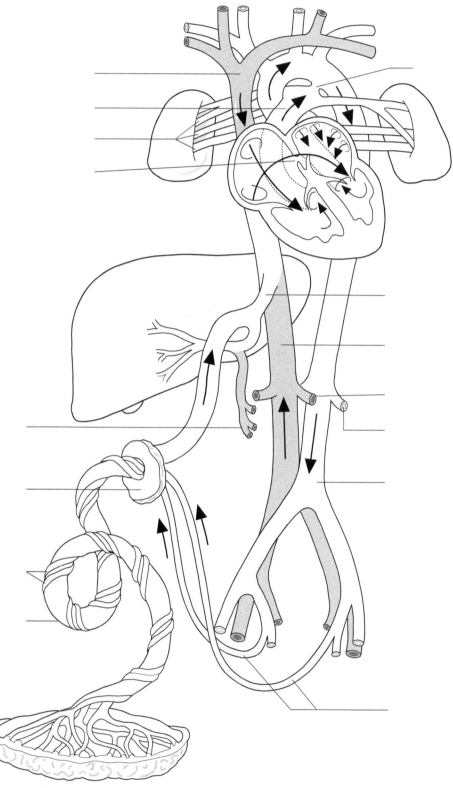

Figure 6.1

Completion

4. Complete the following statements relating to the temporary structures (refer to Figure 6.1).

a. The ductus venosus connects the _____ to the _____.

b. The ductus arteriosus leads from the bifurcation of the _____ to the descending aorta.

c. The foramen ovale is an opening between the _____ and _____ _____

d. The hypogastric arteries branch off from the _____ and become the _____ when they enter the umbilical cord.

5. The flow diagram 6.1 below relates to the flow of blood in the fetal circulation. Complete the diagram to read correctly by removing the incorrect word(s).

Flow diagram 6.1

a. Oxygenated blood from the placenta travels **to/from** the fetus in the **umbilical vein/umbilical arteries**. The **umbilical vein/umbilical arteries** divide**(s)** into two branches: one that supplies the **portal vein/inferior vena cava** in the liver, the other the **ductus venosus/ductus arteriosus** joining the **inferior/superior** vena cava.

↓

b. Most of the oxygenated blood that enters the **right/left** atrium passes across the foramen ovale to the **right/left** atrium and from here into the **left/right** ventricle, and then to the **aorta/pulmonary artery**. The head and **upper/lower** extremities receive about half of the blood supply via the coronary and carotid arteries, and subclavian arteries respectively. The remainder of blood travels in the **descending aorta/inferior vena cava**, mixing with **oxygenated/deoxygenated** blood from the **right/left ventricle**.

↓

c. **Oxygenated/deoxygenated** blood collected from the upper parts of the body returns to the **right/left** atrium in the **inferior/superior** vena cava.

Blood that has entered the **right/left atrium** from the inferior and superior vena cava passes into the **left/right** ventricle. A small amount of blood travels to the lungs in the **pulmonary artery/pulmonary veins** for their development.

↓

d. Most blood passes through the **ductus venosus/arteriosus** into the **ascending/descending** aorta. **Deoxygenated/oxygenated** blood travels back to the placenta via the **internal/external** iliac arteries leading into the hypogastric **arteries/veins** which lead into the umbilical **vein/arteries**.

6. This question relates to the adaptation to extrauterine life. Complete the following statements:

a. The umbilical vein becomes the _____.

b. The ductus venosus becomes the _____.

c. The ductus arteriosus becomes the _____.

d. The hypogastic arteries are known as the _____ except for the first

few centimetres which remain open as the _____.

e. The foramen ovale becomes the _____.

? Multiple choice questions (MCQs)

The following MCQs relate to the embryo/fetal growth and development, fetal circulation and adaptation to extrauterine life.

7. Fetal erythrocytes have a life span of:

   a. 60 days   b. 90 days   c. 120 days   d. 150 days

8. Surfactant:

   a. Is a lipoprotein that reduces surface tension

   b. Is produced by type II alveolar cells

   c. Assists gaseous exchange

   d. All of the above

9. A single umbilical artery at birth is suggestive of abnormalities of the:

   a. Cardiovascular system

   b. Reproductive system

   c. Renal tract

   d. Gastrointestinal tract

10. The neural tube is derived from the:

   a. Ectoderm

   b. Endoderm

   c. Mesoderm

   d. None of the above

11. Fetal haemoglobin (HbF):

   a. Has greater affinity for oxygen than adult haemoglobin (HbA)

   b. Has greater concentrations (18–20 g/dL at term) than adult haemoglobin (HbA)

   c. Is found in the erythrocytes produced by the yolk sac and liver

   d. All of the above

12. In developed countries, the average birth weight is around:

   a. 2800 g

   b. 3000 g

   c. 3400 g

   d. 3800 g

FETAL SKULL

Structures of the fetal skull

✎ Completion

13. The skull is divided into the vault, the base and the face. Complete the missing word/phrases to complete the following descriptions:

a. The base comprises bones that are firmly united to protect _____.

b. The face is composed of _____ small bones which are firmly united and _____

_____.

c. The vault can be described as being a large dome-shaped part above an imaginary line drawn between

the _____ and the _____.

d. What is ossification? It relates to the _____

_____.

e. List three key ossification centres on the skull: i. _____ ii. _____

_____ iii. _____.

f. Define the term suture: _____

_____.

g. Define the term fontanelle: _____

_____.

14. Table 6.3 provides information on the three bones of the vault. Complete the table by providing the missing information.

Table 6.3

	Name the main bone(s) of the vault	Brief description of position	Ossification centre
a.		Lies at the back of the head	
b.		Lie on either side of the skull	
c.		Form the forehead and sinciput	

15. Table 6.4 provides information about the sutures. Complete the table by providing the missing information.

Table 6.4

	Name of suture	Describe position of each suture
a.		Separates the occipital bone from the two parietal bones
b.		Lies between the two parietal bones
c.		Separates the frontal bones from the parietal bones, passing from one temple to the other
d.		Runs between the two halves of the frontal bone

16. Table 6.5 relates to fontanelles. Complete the table by providing the missing information.

Table 6.5

	Name (alternate name)	Shape/size	Position and sutures involved	Closes by:
a.	Posterior fontanelle (alternate name is)			weeks
b.	Anterior fontanelle (alternate name is)			months

  ## Colouring and labelling

17. Figure 6.2 shows the division of the skull. Label and colour the three main divisions – face, vault and base.

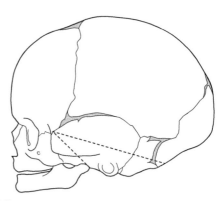

The skull is further separated into regions with important landmarks. During vaginal examinations, the landmarks provide useful information in relation to the position of the fetal head.

Figure 6.2

18. Figure 6.3 presents a view of the fetal head from above with the head partially flexed. Label and colour the figure as listed.

Label and colour

Frontal eminence or boss
Occipital protuberance
Parietal eminence

Label

Anterior fontanelle
Occipital bone
Posterior fontanelle
Frontal bone
Parietal bone

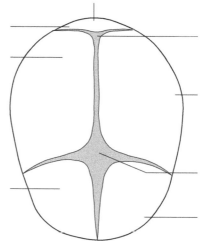

Figure 6.3

Completion

19. Table 6.6 relates to the regions of the fetal head. Complete the table by providing the missing information.

Table 6.6

	Name of region	Position boundaries
a.	Occiput region	Lies between the _____ and _____. The part below the _____ (landmark) is known as sub-occipital region.
b.	Vertex region	This region is bounded by the posterior fontanelle, the _____ and the anterior fontanelle.
c.	Forehead/sinciput region	This region extends from the anterior fontanelle and the _____ to the _____.
d.	Face	Extends from the orbital ridges and the _____ of the _____ to the junction of the chin or _____ (landmark) and the neck. The point between the eyebrows is known as the _____ (landmark).

Landmarks of the fetal skull

 Labelling

20. Figure 6.4 shows the fetal skull regions and landmarks. Label the following structures:

Anterior fontanelle
Mentum
Posterior fontanelle
Occiput region
Frontal bone
Occipital protuberance
Suboccipital region
Glabella
Parietal eminence

Temporal bone
Frontal bone
Parietal bone
Sinciput region
Vertex region
Lambdoidal suture
Coronal suture

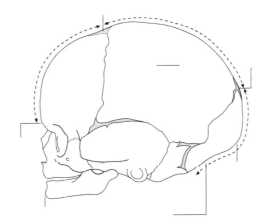

Figure 6.4

Knowledge of the diameters of the skull and diameters of the pelvis are essential to determine the relationship between the fetal head and maternal pelvis during labour.

Completion

21. Table 6.7 relates to the six longitudinal diameters of the fetal skull. Complete the table by providing the missing information.

Table 6.7

	Name of diameter	Areas measured between	(cm)
a.	Sub-occipitobregmatic (SOB)	From below the _____ to the centre of the _____	
b.	Sub-occipitofrontal (SOF)	From below the _____ to the centre of the frontal suture	
c.	_____	From the occipital protuberance to the glabella	
d.	Mentovertical (MV)	From the point of the _____ to the _____ point on the _____ (slightly nearer to the posterior than the anterior fontanelle).	
e.	_____	From the point where the chin joins the neck to the highest point on the vertex	
f.	Sub-mentobregmatic (SMB)	From the point where the chin joins the neck to the centre of the _____.	

22. It is also important to have knowledge of the diameters of the fetal trunk for delivery of the shoulders and breech births.

Describe the following two diameters of the fetal skull (insert measurements):

a. The bisacromial diameter (_____ cm): This is the distance between the _____ on the

_____.

b. Bitrochanteric diameter (_____ cm). This is measured between the greater _____ of the

_____.

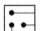 **Labelling**

23. Figure 6.5 shows the transverse diameters of the fetal skull. Label the biparietal diameter and bitemporal diameter and include each measurement (cm).

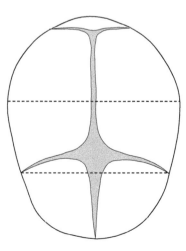

Figure 6.5

Completion

24. The presenting diameters of the fetal head (a longitudinal diameter and transverse diameter) are those that are at right angles to the curve of Carus. The presenting diameters determine the presentation of the fetal head. Complete the following paragraphs about the three presentations of the fetal head by inserting the correct words and numerical values.

a. Vertex presentation:

When the head is well flexed the _____ diameter (_____cm) and the

_____ (_____cm) present. The _____ diameter (_____cm)

distends the vaginal orifice.

When the head is deflexed, the presenting diameters are the _____ (_____cm)

and the _____ (_____cm). This often arises when the occiput is in a posterior

position. If this remains then the _____ diameter (_____cm) distends the

vaginal orifice.

b. Face presentation:

When the head is completely extended the presenting diameters are the

_____ (_____cm) and the _____ (_____cm). The

_____ diameter (_____cm) will distend the vaginal orifice.

c. Brow presentation:

This occurs when the head is partially extended and the _____ diameter (_____cm)

and _____ diameter (_____cm) present. Vaginal birth is unlikely.

Moulding of the fetal skull

 Short answers

25. Complete the following questions:

a. Define the term moulding: _____

_____

b. Why does this happen: _____

_____

_____

Internal structures of the fetal skull

 Labelling

26. Figure 6.6 shows a coronal section through the fetal head to show intracranial membranes and venous sinuses. Label the structures and tissues using the list provided:

Arachnoid mater
Lateral sinus
Pons Varolii
Cerebrum
Medulla oblongata
Sagittal suture
Cerebellum
Parietal bone
Superior sagittal sinus
Falx cerebri
Periosteum
Tentorium cerebelli
Inferior sagittal sinus
Pia mater
Two layers of dura mater

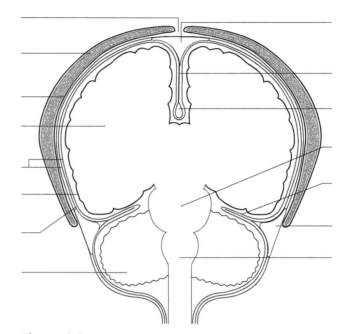

Figure 6.6

27. Figure 6.7 shows intracranial membranes and venous sinuses. Label the structures and tissues using the list provided:

Confluence of sinuses
Inferior sagittal sinus
Superior sagittal sinus
Falx cerebri
Lateral sinus
Tentorium cerebelli
Great cerebral vein
Straight sinus
To internal jugular vein

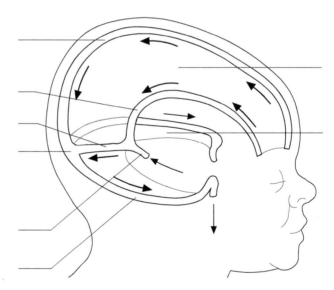

Figure 6.7

? Multiple choice questions (MCQs)

28. The bitrochanteric diameter is the presenting diameter in:

a. Breech presentation

b. Face presentation

c. Brow presentation

d. Vertex presentation

29. The articulation of the clavicles on the sternum may reduce the diameter slightly in the:

a. Mentovertical diameter

b. Bitemporal diameter

c. Bitrochanteric diameter

d. Bisacromial diameter

30. A tear in the tentorium cerebella may result in:

a. Bleeding from the arachnoid mater

b. Bleeding from the great cerebral vein

c. Bleeding from the lateral sinuses

d. None of the above

7 Change and adaptation in pregnancy

The anatomical and physiological adaptations throughout pregnancy affect virtually every body system. It is important to have detailed knowledge of the changes and recognize the variation in timing and intensity of the changes during pregnancy. This chapter will assess your knowledge of changes and adaptations during each stage of pregnancy.

Probable and positive signs of pregnancy

 Completion

1. Signs and symptoms of pregnancy are often enough for a woman to suspect pregnancy. Diagnosis is usually confirmed by the probable signs and positive signs. Complete Table 7.1 by inserting the correct numerical values for time of occurrence from the list provided. You need to identify the hormone.

9–10 days	5.5 weeks	11–12 weeks	20 weeks+
14 days	6–12 weeks+	4–14 weeks	22 weeks+
3–4 weeks+	8 weeks+	16–20 weeks	24 weeks+

Table 7.1

Possible (presumptive) signs	Time of occurrence (weeks)
a. Early breast changes (primigravidae)	
b. Amenorrhoea	4 weeks+
c. Morning sickness	
d. Bladder irritability	
e. Quickening	
Probable signs	**Time of occurrence (day/weeks)**
f. Identify the hormone present: _____	N/A
g. Timing when the hormone is present in blood	
h. Timing when the hormone is present in urine	
i. Changes in skin pigmentation	
Positive signs	**Time of occurrence (weeks)**
j. Gestational sac visible by abdominal ultrasound	
k. Fetal heart sounds by doppler	
l. Fetal heart sounds by fetal stethoscope	
m. Fetal movements palpable	
n. Fetal parts palpated	

The uterus during pregnancy

The uterus plays an essential role in pregnancy by expanding to accommodate the growing fetus and providing support and protection for the fetus, placenta and amniotic fluid. Complete the following activities related to the uterus, vagina and cervix.

True/False

2. Consider the following statements and choose if they are true of false by ticking the appropriate column.

	Statement	True	False
a.	The outer layer of the myometrium lying under the serosal perimetrium is a very thin sheet of smooth muscle.		
b.	The decidua in the cervix and isthmus is more developed than in the corpus.		
c.	Relaxin produced by the decidua plays a part in myometrial quiescence.		
d.	The human myometrium is composed of very well-defined circular and longitudinal layers.		
e.	In the first 12 weeks of pregnancy uterine growth is partly due to hyperplasia and mainly due to hypertrophy.		
f.	The myometrium remains fully quiescent during pregnancy.		
g.	The junctional zone is a separate and distinct functional unit within the uterus lying between the myometrium and deciduas.		
h.	The uterus usually undergoes dextrorotation, possibly because of the rectosigmoid on the right side of the pelvis.		

Completion

3. Complete Table 7.2, which relates to the increase in weight and size of the uterus during pregnancy.

Table 7.2

	Nulliparous	Parous	At term
a. Weight of uterus (g)	60–80	90–100	
b. Size of uterus (cm)	16.8 × 5 × 2.5	9–10	

4. Complete the following statements by inserting the correct word or numerical value from the extended list of options provided:

20	oedema	lowest	endocervical collagen
28	increased vascularity	highest	thin mucus
36	decreased vascularity	endocervical mucosal	hypertrophy
38	internal os	tenacious mucus	

a. The physiological retraction ring develops at the junction between lower and upper segments by _____ weeks' gestation.

b. The fundus reaches the tip of the xyphoid cartilage by _____ weeks' gestation.

c. The isthmus has fully developed into the lower uterine segment by _____ weeks' gestation.

d. Following conception, the cervix becomes softer and cyanosed due to _____ and

_____.

e. In the cervix, the elastin: collagen ratio is greatest in the _____ where the muscle

content is _____.

f. An 'antibacterial plug' develops in the cervix as a result of the _____

cells producing copious amounts of _____.

Changes in the cervix

 Completion

5. Complete the following paragraph about 'ripening' of the cervix by removing the incorrect word so that the paragraph reads correctly:

Cervical ripening involves **inflammatory/stroma** cells but is probably dependent upon **endogenously/exogenously** produced **prostaglandins/oestrogen**. Rearrangement and degradation of **collagen/elastin** fibres creates an **increase/decrease** in the space between them, **shortens/lengthens** them and **increases/decreases** acidic solubility along with **increased/reduced** capacity to **retain/lose** water. The cervix changes to a **soft/firm distensible/rigid** structure with **reduced/increased** resistance to effacement and dilatation.

6. Complete the following terms by inserting the correct word(s) and numerical values from the extended list of options provided:

congestion	fetal heart	oestrogen	vaginal
decreased	Hegar's	Osiander's	4
dilated uterine vessels	increased	placenta	8
discolouration	maternal pulse	progesterone	12
	muffled ocean-like	soft blowing	

   a. The uterine souffle refers to the _____ sound made by the blood passing through

   the _____ and heard distinctly at the lower portion of the uterus. The

   souffle is synchronous with the _____.

   b. The placental souffle refers to the _____ sound of blood coursing through the

   _____. This is synchronous with the _____.

   c. Chadwick's sign refers to violet or dark purplish _____ and _____

   of the vulva and _____ mucous membranes. This is due to _____ vascularity and is

   first detected between the _____ th and _____ th week of pregnancy.

   d. _____ sign refers to the stronger and harder vaginal pulsations in the fornices caused

   by the increased blood supply and enlarged uterine artery.

   e. Leucorrhoea refers to the thick, white_____ discharge and is due to the high

   levels of the hormone _____.

? **Multiple choice questions (MCQs)**

7. In the first 12 weeks of pregnancy, the myometrial cells stretch in length by up to:
   a. 5-fold   b. 10-fold   c. 15-fold   d. 20-fold

8. During pregnancy, the weight of the uterus increases:
   a. 5-fold   b. 10-fold   c. 15-fold   d. 20-fold

9. Comparison between the uterus and fruit has become a fairly reliable way to measure uterine size in early pregnancy. The uterus would feel like a large orange at:

   a. 5 weeks' gestation

   b. 6 weeks' gestation

   c. 8 weeks' gestation

   d. 12 weeks' gestation

10. The uterus is originally pear-shaped. Indicate the weeks of gestation the shape changes to being ovoid:

   a. 12 weeks   b. 16 weeks   c. 20 weeks   d. 24 weeks

11. Which of the following statements relates to Doderlein's bacillus:

   a. This is a normal commensal of the vagina

   b. It metabolizes glycogen to lactic acid

   c. It leads to increased vaginal acidity

   d. All of the above

   e. None of the above

12. In preparation for the distension that occurs in labour, the vaginal walls undergo the following changes:

   a. Mucosa thickens, connective tissue loosens and smooth muscle cells hypertrophy

   b. Mucosa thins, connective tissue loosens and smooth muscle cells hypertrophy

   c. Mucosa thickens, connective tissue and smooth muscle cells remain unchanged

   d. None of the above

Pregnancy is associated with profound but predominantly reversible changes in maternal haemodynamics and cardiac function.

 ## Completion

13. All components of the cardiovascular system (CVS) undergo a degree of adaptation during pregnancy. Table 7.3 presents a summary of the key components of the CVS. Complete the table by removing the incorrect word so that the table reads correctly.

Table 7.3

Key component	Key change in pregnancy
a. Heart	Increases/decreases in size Shifted **upwards/laterally** and to the **left/right**
b. Arteries	Dramatic/minor systemic and pulmonary vasodilation to **decrease/increase** blood flow
c. Capillaries	Increased/decreased permeability
d. Veins	Vasodilation/vasoconstriction and impeded **arterial/venous** return in **upper/lower** extremities
e. Blood	Haemodilution/haemoconcentration, **decreased/increased** capacity for clot formation

14. Table 7.4 relates to the key physiological changes in the CVS during pregnancy. Consider the parameters carefully and complete the missing sections of each column of the table. An incomplete list of options is provided below. Refer to the textbook as required.

Adaptation	Magnitude of change	Timing of peak: average peak values (where relevant)
Minimal – no reduction	10–15%	20 weeks
Reduction and returning to normal by term	21%	28 weeks: 7 L/min
	30–45%	32 weeks: 3850 mL
	35%	1550 mL
	50%	Trimester 1: 90 bpm
		34 weeks

Table 7.4

Parameter	Adaptation (↑,↔,↓, etc.)	Magnitude of change (%, etc.)	Non-pregnant (average value)	Timing of peak: average peak value
Plasma volume			2600 mL	
Red cell mass		N/A	1400 mL	30 weeks:
Total blood volume			mL	32 weeks: 4600 mL
Cardiac output		35–50%	L/min	
Stroke volume	↑	N/A	N/A	
Heart rate			75 bpm	
Systemic vascular resistance			N/A	Trimester 2
Pulmonary vascular resistance	↓		N/A	
Diastolic blood pressure			N/A	24 weeks
Systemic blood pressure		5–10 mmHg	N/A	24 weeks
Serum colloid osmotic pressure			N/A	14 weeks

True/false

15. Consider the following statements and choose if they are true or false by ticking the appropriate column.

	Statement	True	False
a.	The early changes in cardiac output are mainly due to an increase in heart rate in the first trimester.		
b.	As blood volume increases with gestation 10–20% is distributed to the uteroplacental unit.		
c.	While cardiac output is raised, arterial blood pressure is reduced by 10%, therefore resistance to flow is increased.		
d.	The secretion of atrial natriuretic peptide (ANP) is not increased during pregnancy because the ANP-volume is reset during pregnancy.		

 Short answers

16. Complete the following 3 questions related to supine hypotensive syndrome:

a. What is supine hypotensive syndrome?

_____

_____

b. List the six symptoms of supine hypotensive syndrome:

_____

_____

c. What are the potential complications?

_____

_____

 Completion

17. Complete Table 7.5 by providing the missing values:

8 min	10.0–12.0 g/dL	20–25 g/L	4 min
120 × 10⁹L	Usually ≥ 4.5 mmol/L	Usually ≤ 4.5 mmol/L	2.9–6.2 g/L
11.5–16.5 g/dL	25–35 g/L	unchanged	150 × 10⁹L

8 min   10.0–12.0 g/dL   20–25 g/L   4 min

120×10^9L   Usually ≥ 4.5 mmol/L   Usually ≤ 4.5 mmol/L   2.9–6.2 g/L

11.5–16.5 g/dL   25–35 g/L   unchanged 150×10^9L

Table 7.5

Test	Non-pregnant (typical range)	Pregnant (typical range)
Urea (mmol/L)	2–6.5	
Albumin (g/L)	30–48	
Potassium (mmol/L)	3.5–5.3	
Clotting time (min)	12 min	
Fibrinogen (g/L)	1.7–4.1	By term
Haemoglobin (g/dL)		
Alanine transaminase (ALT) (U/L)	6–40	No change
Platelets (x10⁹L)	150–400	Slight decrease

 Short answers

18. The following two questions relate to the apparent anaemia noted during pregnancy:

a. Describe how 'apparent anaemia' occurs during pregnancy: _____

_____

b. Why is 'apparent anaemia' advantageous in a healthy pregnancy?

_____

_____

 True/false

19. Consider the following statements and indicate if they are true or false by ticking the appropriate column:

	Statement	True	False
a.	While total haemoglobin increases the mean haemoglobin concentration falls.		
b.	A haemoglobin level below 10.5 g/100 mL at 28 weeks is normal.		
c.	The majority of increased iron requirements occur in the first trimester.		
d.	Reduced total serum protein content is always a sign of pathology.		
e.	Peripheral oedema in the lower limbs during late pregnancy is a feature of normal pregnancy.		

Completion

20. Consider the following sentences. Complete the statements correctly by removing the incorrect word(s) and values.

   a. The **increased/decreased** tendency to clot is caused by **increases/decreases** in clotting factors and **fibrin/ fibrinogen**.

   b. From **12 weeks'/24 weeks'** gestation there is a **10%/50%** increase in the synthesis of plasma **fibrin/ fibrinogen (factor I/factor X)**.

   c. Coagulation factors VII, VIII and X **increase/decrease** during pregnancy.

21. Table 7.6 provides a summary of changes in the respiratory system. Choose the direction of change by ticking the appropriate column:

Table 7.6

		Increase	Decrease
a.	Oxygen consumption		
b.	Metabolic rate		
c.	Minute volume		
d.	Tidal volume		
e.	Functional residual capacity		
f.	Arterial oxygen tension (PaO$_2$)		
g.	Arterial carbon dioxide tension (PaCO$_2$)		
h.	Arterial pH		

 True/false

22. Consider the following statements and indicate if they are true or false by ticking the appropriate column:

	Statement	True	False
a.	The anterior pituitary gland decreases in size during pregnancy.		
b.	The opioid active form of β endorphin produced by the pituitary is thought to play a major role in raising the maternal threshold for pain and discomfort in the latter stages of pregnancy.		
c.	Glycosuria provides substrates for bacterial growth and can cause asymptomatic bacteruria.		
d.	During pregnancy urinary glucose values can be 10–100-fold greater than non-pregnant values.		
e.	The renin-angiotensin-aldosterone system is important in fluid and electrolyte homeostasis and maintaining blood pressure.		
f.	Pregnancy causes tooth decay. Fetal calcium requirements are drawn from maternal teeth.		
g.	Ptyalism (excessive salivation) is common in pregnancy.		
h.	Gastric emptying of fluids is altered during pregnancy.		
i.	Accelerated starvation refers to a pregnancy induced switch in fuels from glucose to lipids with ketonaemia rapidly appearing.		

 Completion

23. Complete the following paragraph by removing the incorrect word(s) so that the statement reads correctly:

   Dilatation of the ureters, which is rarely present **below/above** the pelvic brim, is possibly due to compression by the enlarging uterus and **ovarian plexus/enlarged kidneys**. The early onset of ureteral dilatation suggests that smooth muscle relaxation, caused by **oestrogen/progesterone**, possibly plays an additional role. The dilatation is more marked on the **right/left** side, due to the cushioning effect of the **ascending/sigmoid** colon on the **right/left** and due to the uterine tendency to **flexion/dextrorotation**.

Short answers

24. This activity relates to the condition known as Pica. Complete the paragraph to provide correct information referring to the textbook if required.

Pica is the _____.

Examples of the substances consumed include clay, _____, _____ or starch.

Pica can cause a number of medical problems, such as nutritional deficiencies, _____

_____ and weight gain.

There are two main viewpoints about the origins of pica practices and these include:

1. _____

2. _____

_____

Completion

25. Consider the following paragraph and remove the incorrect word so that it reads correctly:

In late pregnancy, although basal insulin levels are **elevated/reduced** maternal blood glucose levels are similar to non-pregnant levels and do not **increase/reduce** as rapidly as usual even with **higher/lower** circulating levels of insulin. This diabetogenic state protects the fetus even if the mother is fasting by keeping glucose in the blood and thus available for placental transfer. After a meal, however, the pregnant woman's levels of glucose and insulin are **lower/higher** than those of non-pregnant women and **glycogen/glucagon** is suppressed resulting in **hyper-/hypo-**insulinaemia, **hyper-/hypo-**glycaemia and insulin resistance.

26. Table 7.7 relates to the distribution of maternal and fetal weight gain during pregnancy. Complete the missing information from the list of numerical values (kg) provided below:

0.4 kg   0.9 kg   4.0 kg   7.7 kg

0.7 kg   3.3 kg   4.8 kg

Table 7.7

	Weight gain (kg)
Maternal (64% of total weight gain)	
Uterus	
Breasts	
Fat	
Blood	1.2
Extracellular fluid	1.2
Maternal total	
Fetal (36% of total weight gain)	
Fetus (25%)	
Placenta	
Amniotic fluid	0.8
Total	
Grand Total	12.5

Completion

27. Complete the following paragraph by inserting the missing words from the choices listed below so that the paragraph reads correctly:

oestrogen   relax   progesterone

mobile   softening   relaxin

Relaxation of the pelvic joints is predominantly due to hormonal influences. The hormone

_____ modifies the connective tissue making it more pliable. This causes the joint capsules

to _____, making the pelvic joints _____. The hormone _____ has

the effect of relaxing or weakening the pelvic ligaments. The hormone _____ plays a major

role in the changes, remodelling collagen fibres and _____ pelvic joints and ligaments in

preparation for birth.

Short answers

28. Complete the following questions and activity:

a. What is the recommended pattern for normal weight gain during pregnancy?

_____

b. Which two joints may contribute to the alteration in maternal posture leading to the characteristic 'waddling gait' and back pain of pregnancy?

_____ and _____ joints.

c. What is chloasma (or melasma)? _____

_____

d. What is chloasma (or melasma) also known as? _____

_____.

e. List the other skin changes or skin conditions occurring during pregnancy:

_____

_____

_____.

Changes in the breasts

 Completion

29. Sound knowledge of the changes in the breast is essential. Complete Table 7.8 by providing detailed information of the changes occurring during pregnancy and, where relevant, provide the reason for the change occurring:

Table 7.8

Time	Breast changes	Reason
3–4 weeks		Due to increased blood supply
6–8 weeks		Due to hypertrophy of the alveoli.
8–12 weeks		Hypertrophic sebaceous glands secrete sebum, which keeps the nipple soft. Increased melanin activity.
16 weeks		N/A
Late pregnancy		Progesterone causes the nipple to become more prominent and mobile.

Short answers

30. Complete the following statements/questions:

a. Epulis is a specific _____, which can be caused by advanced

_____.

b. What is leptin?

_____

_____.

c. Where is oxytocin produced in the body?

_____

_____.

d. What are the main effects of oxytocin?

_____

_____.

e. Where is prolactin produced in the body?

_____

_____.

f. What are the main effects of prolactin?

_____

? Multiple choice questions (MCQs)

31. In relation to the circulatory changes in pregnancy, extreme vasodilation is mediated by:

a. Rising pregnancy hormones (particularly progesterone)
b. Rising pregnancy hormones (particularly oestrogen)
c. Circulating nitric oxide
d. a and c
e. b and c

32. During pregnancy, renin and aldosterone activity are both:

a. Increased by oestrogens, progesterone and prostaglandins leading to increased fluid and electrolyte retention
b. Increased by oestrogens, progesterone and prostaglandins leading to decreased fluid and electrolyte retention
c. Increased by oestrogens, progesterone and prostaglandins with no influence on fluid and electrolyte retention
d. None of the above

33. The approximate percentage of women who experience supine hypotensive syndrome during pregnancy is:

a. 10%   b. 20%   c. 30%   d. 50%

34. By the 16th week of pregnancy, renal blood flow has increased by as much as:

a. 20–30%   b. 30–50%   c. 50–60%   d. 70–80%

35. Blood flow in the lower limbs is slowed in late pregnancy by:

a. The enlarging uterus compressing the iliac veins
b. The enlarging uterus compressing the inferior vena cava
c. The hydrodynamic effects of the decreased venous return from the uterus
d. a and b
e. All of the above

36. Normal oxygen consumption at rest is:

    a. 100 mL/min

    b. 150 mL/min

    c. 200 mL/min

    d. 250 mL/min

37. Hyperventilation during pregnancy may lead to mild:

    a. Respiratory alkalosis

    b. Respiratory acidosis

    c. Metabolic alkalosis

    d. Metabolic acidosis

38. Breathlessness (dyspnoea) during pregnancy at rest occurs in:

    a. <10% of women

    b. <20% of women

    c. <45% of women

    d. <60% of women

39. Renin release is stimulated by:

    a. Oestrogens

    b. Relaxin

    c. Higher blood pressure

    d. Decreased levels of plasma and urinary prostaglandins

40. Intestinal absorption of calcium during pregnancy increases:

    a. Two-fold

    b. Ten-fold

    c. Six-fold

    d. Twenty-fold

CHAPTER 8

Antenatal care

Antenatal care refers to the care of pregnant women from the time pregnancy is confirmed until the beginning of labour. This chapter will assess your knowledge of aspects relating to progress in pregnancy, including routine and specialized investigations.

ASSESSMENTS DURING PREGNANCY

First antenatal assessment

Completion

Complete the following activities relating to the first antenatal assessment:

1.

a. What is Naegele's rule? It is _____

_____.

b. If this rule is used then what four assumptions are made:

_____.

_____.

_____.

_____.

2. Body Mass Index (BMI) is the weight in kg divided by the height in m². What is the BMI (cut-off or range) for the following BMI classifications:

a. Underweight: _____ kg/m²   b. Normal: _____ kg/m²

c. Overweight: _____ kg/m²   d. Obese: _____ kg/m²

e. Morbidly obese: _____ kg/m²

Short answers

3. In relation to possible findings on routine urinalysis on the first antenatal visit, complete the following statements:

   a. Ketonuria – ketones are due to the _____.

   Ketonuria may be due to a variety of reasons including _____

   _____.

   b. Proteinuria – protein in the urine may be caused by _____,

   or _____.

4. List the **routine** and possible **other** blood tests offered at the first antenatal appointment:

   a. Routine blood tests: _____

   _____

   _____.

   b. Possible other blood tests: _____

   _____.

Terminology and facts relating to assessment of pregnancy

It is essential that the midwife has detailed knowledge of the terminology and definitions related to assessment of pregnancy. The following activities will test this knowledge.

Completion

5. Complete the following activities a–d.

   a. In relation to 'engagement', define this term: _____

   _____.

   b. Identify the engaging diameter/cm in:

   i. Cephalic presentation: _____ diameter. Measures _____ cm.

   ii. Breech presentation: _____ diameter. Measures _____ cm.

   c. At what gestation does the fetal head normally engage in primigravid women?

   _____.

   d. List the possible causes for non-engagement of the head: _____

   _____

   _____

   _____.

Definitions

6. Complete the following list of definitions:

a. 'Presentation' refers to: _____

_____

b. 'Lie' is: _____

_____

c. 'Attitude' is: _____

d. 'Denominator' means i. _____ and is the ii.

_____

_____

e. 'Position' is: _____

_____

Short answers

7. a. List the types of lie of the fetus (starting with the most commonly occurring):

_____

b. Identify the preferred attitude and <u>describe</u> the fetus with this attitude:

The preferred attitude is _____. The fetus is _____

_____

_____

c. There are three presentations: Complete each of the following statements:

i. In the face presentation the denominator is the _____

ii. In the breech presentation the denominator is the _____

iii. In the vertex presentation the denominator is the _____

Vertex positions

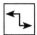 **Matching**

8. Match the vertex positions accurately with the description of the relationship of landmarks to the points on the pelvic brim.

	Description of the occiput in relation to the six points of the pelvis
a.	_____ The occiput points to the symphysis pubis; the sagittal suture is in the anteroposterior diameter of the pelvis.
b.	_____ The occiput points to the left iliopectineal eminence; the sagittal suture is in the right oblique diameter of the pelvis.
c.	_____ The occiput points to the right iliopectineal line midway between the iliopectineal eminence and the sacroiliac joint; the sagittal suture is in the transverse diameter of the pelvis.
d.	_____ The occiput points to the right iliopectineal eminence; the sagittal suture is in the left oblique diameter of the pelvis.
e.	_____ The occiput points to the sacrum; the sagittal suture is in the anteroposterior diameter of the pelvis.
f.	_____ The occiput points to the left sacroiliac joint; the sagittal suture is in the left oblique diameter of the pelvis.
g.	_____ The occiput points to the left iliopectineal line midway between the iliopectineal eminence and the sacroiliac joint; the sagittal suture is in the transverse diameter of the pelvis.
h.	_____ The occiput points to the right sacroiliac joint; the sagittal suture is in the right oblique diameter of the pelvis.

Vertex positions

i.   Right occipitoanterior (ROA)

ii.   Direct occipitoanterior (DOA)

iii. Right occipitolateral (ROL)

iv.   Right occipitoposterior (ROP)

v.   Direct occipitoposterior (DOP)

vi.   Left occipitoanterior (LOA)

vii. Left occipitolateral (LOL)

viii. Left occipitoposterior (LOP)

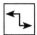 **Labelling**

9. Label the six vertex positions shown in Figure 8.1. Also note the relative frequency of each position.

ROP: _____ %

LOP: _____ %

ROA: _____ %

LOA: _____ %

ROL: _____ %

LOL: _____ %

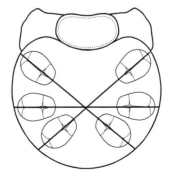

Figure 8.1

Short answers

10. List the three key indicators of fetal wellbeing:

a. _____

b. _____

c. _____

Antenatal tests

Antenatal assessment of the fetus is now a mainstream aspect of care involving both routine and more specialized screening and diagnostic tests for fetal anomaly.

True/false

11. Consider the following statements and decide if they are true or false by ticking the appropriate column.

	Statement	True	False
a.	'False negative rate' from screening tests is the proportion of affected pregnancies that would not be identified as high risk.		
b.	Levels of biochemical markers are never diagnostic for Down syndrome.		
c.	Chorionic villus sampling (CVS) may be performed at any stage before 10 weeks' gestation.		
d.	On ultrasound scan in early pregnancy, the femur is a reliable indicator of gestational age.		
e.	The main advantage of nuchal tube translucency is that it offers an early way of assessing maternal risk for Down syndrome.		
f.	Doppler analysis of the umbilical artery is the only test that improves outcomes in high-risk pregnancies.		
g.	Alphafetoprotein (AFP) is used as a biochemical marker for neural tube defects.		
h.	Alphafetoprotein (AFP) has now been superseded by the use of ultrasound to diagnose neural tube defects.		
i.	Tracheoesophageal fistula is a structural problem readily identified on ultrasound scan.		
j.	Fetuses with excessive growth (macrosomia) are associated with maternal diabetes mellitus.		
k.	In fetal blood sampling, blood can be sampled from the umbilical cord or the intrahepatic umbilical vein.		
L	Raised alphafetoprotein (AFP) levels can be predictive of intrauterine growth restriction and pre-eclampsia.		
m.	Ultrasound waves have not been shown to cause tissue heating.		

 Short answers

Complete the following activities:

12. List the possible reasons for raised AFP levels: _____

_____

13. Provide a comprehensive list of the features examined on detailed ultrasound scan of the fetus:

_____

_____

_____

14. List the potential problems a fetus with assymetrical growth restriction may experience: _____

_____

15. What is nuchal translucency (NT)? _____

_____

16. Name the two main rapid diagnostic techniques: _____

_____

17. Name two new and emerging technologies for fetal investigations: _____

_____

 ## Multiple choice questions (MCQs)

18. Examples of diagnostic tests include:

   a. Ultrasound scan

   b. Chorionic villus sampling

   c. Amniocentesis

   d. All of the above

19. The incidence of mothers with raised AFP levels is:

   a. <1%   b. 2%   c. 5%   d. 7%

20. Increased nuchal translucency is associated with:

   a. Genetic disorders

   b. Structural disorders

   c. Chromosomal disorders

   d. a and c

   e. All of the above

21. Gestational age is primarily assessed by biparietal diameter:

   a. Before 8 weeks' gestation

   b. Between 8 and 12 weeks' gestation

   c. After 13 weeks' gestation

   d. In late pregnancy

22. Detailed fetal anomaly screening ultrasound scan is usually performed between:

   a. 10–12 weeks' gestation

   b. 14–16 weeks' gestation

   c. 18–20 weeks' gestation

   d. 22–24 weeks' gestation

23. Gestational age is accurately assessed by crown-rump length (CRL):

   a. Before 13 weeks' gestation

   b. In early second trimester

   c. In mid pregnancy

   d. In late pregnancy

9 Problems in pregnancy

> The first section of this chapter will focus on abnormalities and problems specifically experienced in the first 20 weeks of pregnancy. The later section will deal with problems experienced in the second half of pregnancy. This chapter will assess your knowledge of abnormalities and problems occurring during pregnancy.

PROBLEMS IN EARLY PREGNANCY

 Definition

The following activities relate to problems in early pregnancy.

1. Complete the following definitions:

a. 'Implantation bleeding' relates to _____

_____

b. 'Spontaneous miscarriage' is the _____

_____

c. 'Recurrent miscarriage' is defined as _____

_____

d. 'Ectopic pregnancy' refers to _____

_____

Early pregnancy loss

 Short answers

2. No definite cause can be found for many cases of miscarriage. Name the known causes:

_____

_____

_____

3. Spontaneous miscarriages progress through a number of stages with the clinical symptoms of vaginal bleeding and abdominal pain. Name the different stages (or types) of miscarriage: _____

_____

_____

4. Infection may be introduced into the genital tract during the process of miscarriage/therapeutic termination:

   a. List the additional clinical findings found if infection is present: _____

_____

   b. What are the manifestations/complications of overwhelming infection: _____

_____

_____

   c. Name two common organisms which invade the uterine cavity: _____

_____

Ectopic pregnancy

Labelling

5. Figure 9.1 shows the site of implantation of ectopic pregnancy. Label the sites.

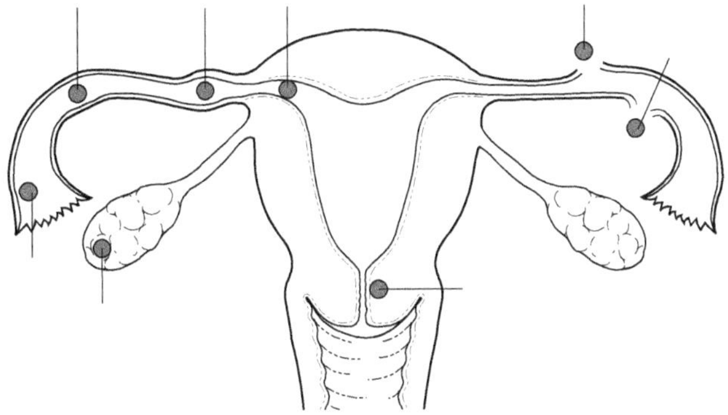

Figure 9.1

Completion and short answers

6. In relation to the clinical 'acute' presentation of ectopic pregnancy:

   a. Identify and detail the classical pattern of symptoms:

_____

_____

_____

   b. Detail the clinical findings:

_____

_____

_____

Trophoblastic disease

✎ Completion

7. The following paragraph relates to trophoblastic disease. Complete the paragraphs to read correctly by filling in the missing words from the extended list below.

anaemia	early weeks	missed	second half of
bleeding	first half of	ovarian cysts	smaller
bloated	hyperemesis	pain	snowstorm
constipation	larger	pre-eclampsia	threatened
complete	late	pyrexia	

Molar pregnancy most commonly presents with _____ in the _____

pregnancy. It is usually diagnosed initially as a _____ miscarriage. The uterus is

_____ than dates in about half of the cases. On ultrasound examination a

'_____' appearance usually suggests molar disease. Associated conditions include: unexplained

_____, severe _____, _____ and _____.

Nausea and vomiting

8. Complete the following statements related to nausea and vomiting in early pregnancy:

a. Hyperemesis gravidarum is defined as being _____

_____

b. The clinical features of dehydration include _____

_____

c. Prolonged vomiting can be associated with other life-threatening complications including _____

_____

9. Name other possible causes of abdominal pain in early pregnancy related to the reproductive tract (excluding miscarriage, ectopic pregnancy):

_____

_____

Miscellaneous activities related to problems in early pregnancy

 True/false and pot luck

10. Consider the following statements and decide whether they are true or false by ticking the appropriate column.

	Statement	True	False
a.	Ectopic pregnancy is the commonest cause of direct maternal death in early pregnancy		
b.	Cervical excitation refers to the tenderness of the cervix when moved		
c.	The commonest site of extrauterine implantation is the uterine tube, usually in the region of the isthmus		
d.	Trophoblastic disease is always benign		
e.	Symptoms of pain, bleeding and amenorrhoea may be absent in the subacute phase of ectopic pregnancy		
f.	The uterus is said to be retroverted where the long axis of the uterus and the axis of the vagina is >180°		

 Multiple choice questions (MCQs)

11. The incidence of vaginal bleeding in pregnancy prior to 20 weeks' gestation is:

   a. 10%   b. 25%   c. 30%   d. 40%

12. The incidence of ectopic pregnancies in the UK is:

   a. 1 in 50 pregnancies

   b. 1 in 100 pregnancies

   c. 1 in 500 pregnancies

   d. 1 in 1000 pregnancies

13. The overall accuracy of clinical diagnosis of ectopic pregnancy is:

   a. 10%   b. 25%   c. 50%   d. 75%

PROBLEMS IN LATE PREGNANCY

  Definitions and short answers

Complete the following definitions, statements and activities.

14. a. Pelvic girdle pain (PGP) is also known as _____ (_____).

   It is characterized by _____

   _____.

   This is brought about by several factors including _____

   _____

   _____.

   It affects 1 in _____ women.

   b. Antepartum haemorrhage refers to _____

   _____.

c. The condition known as placenta praevia refers to _____

_____

_____.

d. Placenta abruption is defined as _____

_____.

e. Blood loss from a placental abruption may be defined as being _____,

_____, or _____ haemorrhages.

Short answers

15. Describe what is meant by the term 'Couvelaire uterus' including the signs and symptoms:

_____

_____

_____

_____

_____

Classification of placenta praevia

Completion

16. Consider the following statements and decide which of the most appropriate classification of placenta praevia the statement applies to by ticking the relevant column.

	Statement	Type 1	Type 2	Type 3	Type 4
a.	The placenta is located over the internal os but not centrally.				
b.	This is also described as being a marginal placenta praevia.				
c.	The placenta is located centrally over the internal os.				
d.	Fetal hypoxia is more likely to be present than maternal shock.				
e.	Caesarean section is essential to save the lives of mother and baby.				
f.	The majority of the placenta is in the upper segment.				
g.	Vaginal birth is not appropriate because the placenta precedes the fetus.				
h.	Blood loss is usually moderate, although the conditions of the mother and fetus may vary.				
i.	The placenta is partially located in the lower segment near the internal os.				
j.	Blood loss is usually mild and the mother and fetus remain in good condition.				
k.	Bleeding is likely to be severe particularly when the lower segment stretches and the cervix begins to efface and dilate in late pregnancy.				
l.	Vaginal birth is possible.				
m.	Vaginal birth is possible, particularly if the placenta is anterior.				
n.	Torrential haemorrhage is likely.				

True/false and pot luck

17. Consider the following statements and decide if they are true or false by ticking the appropriate column.

	Statement	True	False
a.	As the uterus grows during pregnancy it usually rotates to the right by no more than 40°.		
b.	On no account must any vaginal or rectal examination be performed to assess a woman with an antepartum haemorrhage.		
c.	In placental abruption, blood retained behind the placenta may be forced into the myometrium.		
d.	Uterine apoplexy is another term for placenta praevia (stage 4).		
e.	Placenta accreta is a complication in 50% of women with placenta praevia.		
f.	Pituitary necrosis is also known as Sheehan's syndrome. This is a serious complication of haemorrhage.		

Blood clotting

Completion

18. Consider the key choices of words provided below. Complete the following paragraphs related to blood clotting using the relevant word (some words may be used more than once).

clot	fibrinolysis	clotting factors	fibrin
plasma	thrombin	coagulation mechanism	fibrinogen
platelets	thromboplastin	heparin	prothrombin

Normal blood clotting occurs in three main stages:

1. When tissues are damaged and _____ breakdown, _____ is released;

2. In the presence of calcium ions, _____ leads to the conversion of

_____ into _____;

3. _____ is a proteolytic (protein-splitting) enzyme that converts _____ into fibrin.

_____ forms a network of long-sticky strands that entrap blood cells to form a _____. The

coagulated material contracts and exudes a serum which is _____ depleted of _____

_____. The _____ is normally held at bay by the presence of

_____ which is produced in the liver.

_____ is the breakdown of fibrin and occurs in response to the presence of clotted blood.

Coagulation will continue unless _____ takes place.

Disseminating intravascular coagulation

Disseminating intravascular coagulation (DIC) is a situation of inappropriate coagulation which leads to consumption of clotting factors. As a result, clotting fails and triggers widespread clotting with the formation of microthrombin throughout the circulation.

Short answer

19. Identify obstetric situations/events that may trigger DIC during pregnancy:

_____

_____

_____

? **Multiple choice questions (MCQs)**

20. Which of the following statements about placenta praevia is correct?

   a. Complicates 3–6 of every 1000 pregnancies

   b. Has a raised incidence in women who smoke

   c. Has an increased incidence in women who have had a previous caesarean section

   d. Is more common in multigravidae

   e. All of the above

21. Which of the following statements about placental abruption is correct?

   a. Occurs in 5% of all pregnancies

   b. Always involves vaginal bleeding

   c. Partial separation of the placenta causes bleeding from the maternal venous sinuses in the placental bed

   d. Is not associated with a reduction in uterine size

   e. All of the above

22. DIC results in situations involving intrauterine fetal death retained in utero for longer than 3 weeks due to the dead fetal tissue releasing:

   a. Thromboplastin   b. Thrombin   c. Fibrin   d. Heparin   e. None of the above

Hepatic disorders and jaundice in pregnancy

 True/false

23. Complete the following activity related to hepatic disorders and jaundice in pregnancy. Consider the statements and choose if they are true or false by ticking the appropriate column.

	Statement	True	False
a.	Intrahepatic cholestasis of pregnancy usually begins in the third trimester.		
b.	There are no known associated risks with intrahepatic cholestasis of pregnancy.		
c.	Acute fatty liver of pregnancy is a rare condition resulting in death to mother and fetus if a diagnosis is not made or correct treatment given.		
d.	Fever is common in viral hepatitis.		
e.	Hepatitis A occurs as an acute infection spread mainly by ingesting water contaminated with faecal matter.		
f.	In hepatitis B, the risk of liver damage is considered to be greater in the fetus than the mother through transplacental passage of the virus and particularly through blood and body fluids at birth.		
g.	Hepatitis C virus is easier to acquire than hepatitis B and carries a lower risk of chronic liver disease.		
h.	Generalized pruritus may be a symptom of hepatic related conditions and women should always be referred to a medical practitioner.		

Miscellaneous related problems

✎ Completion

24. Complete the following statements:

    a. Normal amniotic fluid increases in amount until 38 weeks when it is around _____ L.

    b. Normal amniotic fluid is around _____ mL at term.

    c. Chronic hydramnios has a gradual onset usually starting from about _____ weeks' gestation.

    d. Acute hydramnios usually occurs around _____ weeks' gestation and is frequently associated with

        _____ or _____.

    e. Oligohydramnios is an abnormally small amount of amniotic fluid which at term may be

        _____–_____ mL.

❓ Multiple choice questions (MCQs)

25. Pemphigoid gestationis (herpes gestationis) is a:

    a. Condition related to herpes virus

    b. Disease not specific to pregnancy

    c. Condition initiated by a maternal autoimmune response to paternal antigens

    d. Skin disorder only affecting the face

    e. All of the above

26. It is estimated that the incidence of pregnancies complicated by cancer is:

    a. 1 in 1000–1500 pregnancies

    b. 1 in 3000–5000 pregnancies

    c. 1 in 5000–7000 pregnancies

    d. 1 in 8000–10000 pregnancies

27. The most common two causes of cancer during pregnancy are:

    a. Cervix and ovary

    b. Breast and leukemia

    c. Melanoma and colorectum

    d. Leukemia and lymphoma

28. Pre-term pre-labour rupture of membranes (PPROM):

    a. Affects 10% of all pregnancies

    b. Occurs before 37 completed weeks' gestation

    c. Is not associated with cervical incompetence

    d. All of the above

    e. None of the above

10 Conditions in pregnancy

> The chapter combines a variety of topics including medical and hypertensive disorders in pregnancy, sexually transmitted infections of the reproductive tract and multiple births. This chapter will provide activities to assess your knowledge of related aspects to these topic areas.

MEDICAL AND HYPERTENSIVE DISORDERS IN PREGNANCY

The physiological changes during pregnancy already have a profound impact on the body systems. This may be further complicated by a range of medical disorders and conditions the woman may already experience.

Diabetes mellitus

 Completion

1. The following activities relate to diabetes mellitus which is a chronic and progressive disorder.

   a. Complete the following paragraphs by inserting the correct word(s) from the extended list provided.

carbohydrates	glycogen	kidney disease	peripheral arterial disease
coronary heart disease	glucagon	loss of vision	protein
excessive thirst	hyperglycaemia	nerve damage	proteinuria
excessive urinary excretion	hypoglycaemia	metabolic	unexplained weight gain
glycosuria	insulin	metabolism	unexplained weight loss

   The term 'diabetes mellitus' describes a _____ disorder that affects the normal

   _____ of _____. It is characterized by _____ and

   _____ resulting from defects in _____ secretion or action, or both. The classics signs

   and symptoms are _____

   _____.

   The long term effects include_____

   _____

   _____.

b. Complete the following statements by inserting the correct word(s) from the extended list of options provided, with a few words being used more than once.

alpha	carbohydrate intolerance	hypoglycaemia	lack of physical activity	pancreas
beta	defect	insulin	obesity	glycogen
carbohydrate tolerance	hyperglycaemia	islets of Langerhans	pregnancy	glucagon

Classification	Statement
Type 1 diabetes	This occurs when _____ cells in the _____ located in the _____ are destroyed, stopping the production of _____.
Type 2 diabetes	This results from a _____ in the action of _____. The risk of developing this type of diabetes increases with age, _____, and _____.
Gestational diabetes (GDM)	This is defined as _____ resulting in _____ of variable severity. Onset or first recognition occurs during _____.

c. Consider the extended list of numerical values below. Complete the following statements by matching the correct value from the extended list provided noting that some values may be used more than once.

1.2   2.2   3.2   4.1   5.1   6.1   7.0   7.8

8.0   8.5   10.0   15.0   20.0   25.0   30.0

i.   Normal fasting blood glucose level <_____ mmol/L

ii. Hypoglycaemia is defined as a blood glucose level <_____ mmol/L

iii. Severe hyperglycaemia is a blood glucose level of >_____ mmol/L

iv. Impaired glucose tolerance is categorized as slightly raised post-meal blood glucose levels of >_____ mmol/L

v.   Impaired fasting glycaemia refers to blood glucose levels within the range >_____ mmol/L and <_____ mmol/L

Miscellaneous medical conditions during pregnancy

Completion

2. Anaemia is a reduction in the oxygen carrying capacity of the blood. List the signs and symptoms of anaemia:

signs: _____ symptoms: _____

_____

_____

True/false

3. Consider the following statements and decide if they are true or false by ticking the appropriate column.

	Statement	True	False
a.	Absorption of iron is inhibited by tea and coffee.		
b.	Many of the symptoms of normal pregnancy resemble those of heart disease.		
c.	The onset of primary tuberculosis (TB) is often insidious and the symptoms non-specific.		
d.	The most common cause of hyperthyroidism in pregnancy is autoimmune thyroiditis (Hashimoto's disease).		
e.	There is a physiological increase in serum folate levels during pregnancy.		
f.	The cause of folic acid deficiency anaemia is never due to a reduced dietary intake.		
g.	Alcohol may interfere with the utilization of folic acid.		
h.	A deficiency of vitamin B12 also produces a megaloblastic anaemia.		
i.	Haemoglobinopathies describe inherited conditions where the haemoglobin is abnormal.		
j.	Women who suffer from spherocytosis may have had a splenectomy.		
k.	Many autoimmune diseases are more prevalent in women between puberty and the menopause.		
L	Grave's disease is the most common cause of hyperthyroidism in pregnancy.		

 Multiple choice question (MCQs)

4. Marfan's syndrome is a connective tissue disease caused by:

  a. Autosomal dominant defect on chromosome 15

  b. Autosomal recessive defect on chromosome 15

  c. Autosomal dominant defect on chromosome 10

  d. Autosomal recessive defect on chromosome 10

5. Aortic dissection (acute) may occur in pregnancy in association with:

  a. Severe hypertension

  b. Co-arctation of the aorta

  c. Connective tissue disease (e.g. Marfan's syndrome)

  d. All of the above

  e. None of the above

6. Severe anaemia is defined as:

  a. Hb level <9 g/dL

  b. Hb level <6 g/dL

  c. Hb level <7 g/dL

  d. Hb level <8 g/dL

7. For women with iron deficiency anaemia, first line treatment is oral iron preparations of:

  a. 120–240 mg/day

  b. 200–300 mg/day

  c. 300–400 mg/day

  d. 400–500 mg/day

8. Very severe anaemia is defined as:

   a. Hb level <4 g/dL

   b. Hb level <3 g/dL

   c. Hb level <5 g/dL

   d. Hb level <6 g/dL

9. Sickle cells have an increased fragility and shortened lifespan of:

   a. 10 days   b. 13 days   c. 17 days   d. 21 days

Hypertensive disorders of pregnancy represent the most significant complication of pregnancy. The following related activities will test knowledge of these disorders.

Hypertension during pregnancy

 Completion

10. Describe (in line with the PRECOG 2004) the following main categories of hypertension during pregnancy by inserting the missing words in the following table from the options provided. Some words and numerical values may be used more than once.

before	headache	low	placenta	seizures
cerebral	hypertension	kidney	proteinuria	upper abdominal
diastolic	liver	multi-system	raised	90
20	30	110	160	1+
2+	3+			

	Category	Detailed description
a.	Pre-existing or chronic hypertension	This is known as hypertension _____ pregnancy or a _____ blood pressure of _____ mmHg pre-pregnancy or before _____ weeks' gestation.
b.	New, gestational or pregnancy-induced hypertension	This is the development of hypertension at or after _____ weeks' gestation when the woman's _____ blood pressure was <_____ mmHg before _____ weeks' gestation. There are no other signs of pre-eclampsia.
c.	New proteinuria	This is the presence of _____ defined as _____ (300 mg/L or more) on dipstick testing, a protein-creatinine ratio of ≥_____ mg/mmol on a random sample, or a urine _____ excretion of ≥300 mg/24 hours.
d.	Pre-eclampsia	This is diagnosed on the basis of new hypertension with significant _____ at or after _____ weeks' gestation. Pre-eclampsia is a _____ disorder, which can affect the _____, _____, brain, and other organs. In the absence of _____, pre-eclampsia is suspected when _____ is accompanied by symptoms including _____, blurred vision, _____ pain, or altered biochemistry: specifically _____ urates, _____ platelet counts and abnormal _____ enzyme levels. These signs and symptoms together with blood pressure >_____ mmHg systolic or >_____ mmHg diastolic and proteinuria of _____ or _____ on a dipstick, demonstrate the more severe form of pre-eclampsia.
e.	Eclampsia	This is defined as the new onset of _____ during pregnancy or postpartum, unrelated to other _____ pathological conditions, in a woman with pre-eclampsia.
f.	Superimposed pre-eclampsia	The development of pre-eclampsia in women with pre-existing _____ and/or pre-existing _____.

11. Complete the following activity by removing the incorrect word so that the alterations in the haematological and biochemical parameters (suggesting the onset of pre-eclampsia) read correctly.

    a. Haemoglobin – **increased/decreased** levels

    b. Haematocrit – **increased/decreased** levels

    c. Platelet count <150 × 10^9/L – known as **thrombocytopenia/hypovolaemic**

    d. Clotting times – **prolonged/reduced**

    e. Serum creatinine (>90 mm/L) and urea levels – **raised/lowered**

Normal blood values in pregnancy

12. Consider the following extended selection of numerical values below. From this selection complete the following table in relation to the range in normal blood values in pregnancy.

33–39%	150–$400 \times 10^9/L$	3.63–4.23 g/L
36–42%	100–$250 \times 10^9/L$	2.53–3.10 g/L
28–32%	300–$500 \times 10^9/L$	4.23–512 g/L

Full blood count	Range	Full blood count	Range
Haemoglobin	11.1–12 g/dl	Platelets	_____ × 10⁹/L
Haematocrit	_____ %	Fibrinogen	_____ g/L

True/false

13. Consider the following statements related to hypertensive disorders of pregnancy and choose if they are true or false.

	Statement	True	False
a.	The placenta is thought to be the primary cause of pre-eclampsia.		
b.	Damage to the endothelial cells with widespread inflammation will decrease the production of thromboxane (Tx), a potent vasoconstrictor.		
c.	Where there is a large placental mass, hypertensive disorders are more likely to occur.		
d.	The coagulation cascade is activated due to disruption of the vascular endothelium and vasoconstriction.		
e.	Thrombocytopenia results from the consumption of platelets.		
f.	In the kidneys, hypertension leads to vasospasm of the afferent arterioles resulting in decreased renal.		
g.	Renal damage is reflected in increased creatinine clearance and reduced serum creatinine and uric acid levels.		
h.	In a severe case of oedema in the liver cells, swelling causes lower abdominal pain and can lead to intracapsular haemorrhages.		
i.	In hypertensive encephalopathy the autoregulation of cerebral blood flow is disrupted resulting in vasospasm, cerebral oedema and blood clot formation.		
j.	Women with pre-eclampsia are hypovolaemic.		

HELLP syndrome

Completion

14. Complete the following activities in relation to the condition known as HELLP syndrome.

a. What does the abbreviation HELLP stand for?

H: _____   EL: _____   LP: _____

_____   _____

b. Complete the following paragraph by inserting the missing words and numerical values from the extended list provided.

abruptio	liver	nausea	upper	34
full blood count	malaise	renal failure	vomiting	30
intravascular coagulation	maternal blood pressure	tenderness	32	48
pancreas	lower	72	12	20

HELLP syndrome typically manifests itself between _____ and _____ weeks' gestation. Of all cases,

_____% will occur postpartum with the onset typically being within _____ hours following birth. Women

with HELLP syndrome will often complain of several symptoms including _____,

_____ and _____, _____ abdominal pain with _____.

Some women will experience non-specific viral-like symptoms. Investigations include _____

_____, platelet count and liver function tests. These should be carried out irrespective of _____

_____ readings. Serious maternal complications include i. _____

placentae, ii. disseminated _____, iii. eclampsia, iv. acute

_____ and v. sub-capsular haematoma of the _____.

Eclampsia

15. Complete the following table relating to the signs of impending eclampsia by inserting the missing word(s) or choosing the correct word(s).

Sign or symptom	Statement
Blood pressure	There is a sharp **rise/fall** in BP.
Headache	This is described as being **severe/dull** and **intermittent/persistent**. It is usually located in the **frontal/occipital** region. This is due to **cerebral vasospasm/dehydration**.
Level of consciousness	The woman is **awake/drowsy** and **alert/confused**. This is due to **cerebral vasospasm/dehydration**.
Visual	There are visual disturbances such as _____ and _____. This is due to **cerebral vasospasm/dehydration**.
Urinary output	Output is _____. There may be an increase in _____. This woman is in **hepatic/renal** failure.
Abdominal pain	There is **upper/lower** abdominal pain. This is due to **liver/pulmonary oedema**. The woman may also have nausea and _____.

？ Multiple choice questions (MCQs)

16. Significant proteinuria is defined as being urine protein excretion:

a. ≥ 100 mg/24 hours

b. ≥ 200 mg/24 hours

c. ≥ 300 mg/24 hours

d. ≥ 400 mg/24 hours

17. Mean arterial blood pressure (MAP) is:

a. Half the systolic blood pressure plus the diastolic pressure divided by 3.

b. Systolic blood pressure plus twice the diastolic pressure divided by 3.

c. Diastolic blood pressure plus half the systolic blood pressure divided by 2.

d. Systolic blood pressure minus the diastolic blood pressure multiplied by 2.

18. What is the MAP if the systolic pressure is 128 mmHg and the diastolic pressure is 80 mmHG?

   a. 74 mmHg

   b. 48 mmHg

   c. 93 mmHg

   d. 96 mmHg

SEXUALLY TRANSMITTED INFECTIONS

 Matching

19. Consider the key choices of infections provided and complete the following activity by matching these to the key mode of transmission.

Genital, bacterial and viral infections of the reproductive tract			
a. Human immunodeficiency virus (HIV)	b. Trichomiasis	c. Human cytomegalovirus (HMVC)	d. Genital warts
e. Group B streptococcus (GBS)	f. Gonorrhoea	g. Hepatitis B virus (HBV)	h. Vulvovaginal candidiasis
i. Syphilis	j. Chlamydia	Herpes simplex virus (HSV) k. Type 1 HSV-1, l. Type 2 HSV-2	m. Bacterial vaginosis (BV)

Key mode of transmission	Infection (a–m)
i. Confirmed to be transmitted sexually	
ii. Associated with close contact with sexual partner/increased sexual activity	
iii. Not associated with sexual transmission	

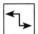 **Matching**

20. Using the extended selection of infections listed above complete the following table by matching the statement accurately to the related type of infection.

	Statement	Infection
i.	It is one of the most common sexually transmitted infections. The infection may be acquired perinatally and occurs in 5% of babies born to infected mothers. A classic frothy yellow-green discharge occurs in 10–30% of women.	
ii.	This infection is the most common cause of vaginal discharge. It is associated with sexual activity and often co-exists with other sexually transmitted infections.	
iii	Factors that predispose to this infection include: changes to vaginal flora (e.g. antibiotics, spermacides), poor diabetic control, pregnancy and immunosuppressant disease.	
iv.	This infection may cause systemic disease and arthritis.	
v.	This is an acute and chronic infection that can be transmitted transplacentally to the fetus from 9th week of gestation onwards. It is classified into early infective stage and late non-infective stage.	
vi.	This infection is the leading cause of serious neonatal infection in the UK.	
vii.	This infection belongs to a family of DNA viruses that cause infection of the liver.	
viii.	This infection is caused by human papillomavirus (HPV).	
ix.	Serotypes (A, B & C) of this infection cause trachoma and blindness. Serotypes (L1 – L3) cause genital disease lymphogranuloma venereum.	

MULTIPLE PREGNANCIES

 Completion

21. Complete the following definitions:

   a. Monozygotic twins develop from the fusion of _____

   _____.

b. Dizygotic twins develop from _____

_____.

c. Superfecundation is the term used when twins are conceived from _____

_____.

d. Superfetation is the term used for twins conceived as a result of _____

_____.

e. Zygosity means determining whether or not twins are _____

_____.

Short answers

22. Detail the physiological characteristics of:

a. Monozygote twins _____

_____

_____

_____.

b. Dizygote twins: _____

_____.

True/false

23. Consider the following statements and decide if they are true or false by ticking the appropriate column.

	Statement	True	False
a.	Twin babies with a single outer membrane (chorion) they must be monochorionic and monozygotic.		
b.	At birth dichorionic twins have a greater weight variation than monochorionic twins.		
c.	Both monozygotic and dizygotic twins can have separate placentae, two chorions and two amnions.		
d.	Both monozygotic and dizygotic twins can have fused placentae, two chorions and two amnions.		
e.	Only monozygotic twins can have a single placenta, one chorion and two amnions.		
f.	In both monozygotic and dizygotic twins, the type of placenta produced is determined immediately at conception.		
g.	'Lambda sign' relates to the tongue of placental tissue between the two chorions seen on ultrasound scan.		

Multiple choice questions (MCQs)

24. The incidence of twin births in the UK is:

    a. 1 in 44 births

    b. 1 in 50 births

    c. 1 in 66 births

    d. 1 in 84 births

25. The chance of any woman having monozygotic twins is:

    a. 1 in 250–300

    b. 1 in 350–400

    c. 1 in 500–800

    d. 1 in 900–1200

26. There is a familial history of:

    a. Both monozygotic and dizygotic twins

    b. Monozygotic twins on the female side

    c. Monozygotic twins on the male side

    d. Dizygotic twins on the male side

    e. Dizygotic twins on the female side

27. In relation to polyhydramnios which of the following statements is correct:

    a. Polyhydramnios is associated with fetal abnormalities

    b. Polyhydramnios is associated with twin to twin transfusion syndrome (TTTS)

    c. Acute polyhydramnios may occur in pregnancy as early as 16 weeks' gestation

    d. All of the above

    e. None of the above

This chapter focuses on the physiology of first and second stage of labour. The transition from pregnancy to labour is a sequence of events that often begins gradually. The range of activities will test your knowledge of terminology and the physiological and physical developments related to these stages.

FIRST STAGE OF LABOUR

Labour is a continuous and dynamic process and there is now more acknowledgement that there are not just three clear phases of normal labour. However, for the purpose of this workbook, the traditional definitions of labour will be used until current uncertainty surrounding this area results in further clearly defined parameters.

Stages of labour

 Matching

1. Table 11.1 provides statements about labour as defined by NICE (2007). Complete the table by ticking the appropriate column each statement refers to.

Table 11.1

	Statement	Latent first stage	Established first stage	Passive second stage	Active second stage
a.	There is active maternal effort following confirmation of full dilatation of the cervix in the absence of expulsive contractions.				
b.	The period of time is not necessarily continuous when there are painful contractions.				
c.	There is some cervical change, including cervical effacement and dilatation up to 4 cm.				
d.	There is progressive cervical dilatation from 4 cm.				
e.	There are expulsive contractions with a finding of full dilatation of the cervix.				
f.	There is a finding of full dilatation of the cervix prior to involuntary expulsive contractions.				
g.	The baby is visible.				
h.	There are regular painful contractions.				

 Matching and completion

2. Complete the following statements related to the first stage of labour in Table 11.2 by matching them correctly to the list of terms provided.

a. Bandl's ring   b. Cervical dilatation   c. Cervical effacement   d. Formation of forewaters

e. Lower uterine segment   f. Operculum   g. Polarity   h. Retraction

i. Retraction ring   j. Show   k. Spurious labour   l. Upper uterine segment

Table 11.2

	Statements
i.	This refers to the process leading to the inclusion of the cervical canal into the lower uterine segment.
ii.	Dilatation and effacement of the cervix are absent.
iii.	Muscle fibres retain some of the shortening of contraction.
iv.	This term is used to describe the ridge formed between the upper and lower uterine segments in uncomplicated labour.
v.	This refers to the blood-stained mucoid discharge seen by the woman in early labour and the small loss of bright red blood during the transitional phase.
vi.	This is caused by the chorion detaching from the uterine segment as it forms and stretches causing the loosened part of the amniotic sac to bulge downwards into the internal os.
vii.	This exaggerated ridge between the upper and lower segments becomes visible above the symphysis in mechanically obstructed labour when the lower segment thins abnormally.
viii.	This thick, muscular portion of the uterus is mainly concerned with contraction and retraction.
ix.	This thinner portion of the uterus is formed of the isthmus and the cervix.
x.	This term refers to the cervical plug during pregnancy.
xi.	This occurs as a result of uterine action and the counterpressure applied by the intact bag of membranes or the presenting part, or both.
xii	This term describes the neuromuscular harmony between the two poles of the uterus throughout labour.

Fundal dominance

  Colouring and labelling

3. Figure 11.1 presents a series of diagrams to show fundal dominance during uterine contractions. Starting on the top row and working left to right over the seven diagrams, use 3 colour shades (strong, medium and weak) to show fundal dominance and the spread of the contraction over the uterus. Using the lists provided, colour and label the figure.

Colour (insert each shade in the figure into the relevant box indicating strength of contraction below)

Strong   Medium   Weak

Label

Contraction: starting → spreading → height of contraction → fading → uterus retracted.

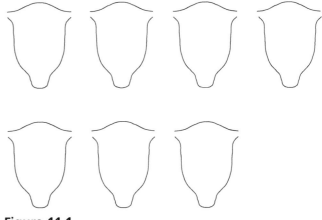

Figure 11.1

Vaginal examination

 Completion

4. Table 11.3 by filling in the missing words relating to the indications to perform vaginal examination from the list provided. A few words may be used more than once.

amniotic sac	delay	full dilatation	progress
axis	engaged	ill-fitting	ruptured
cervix	fetal heart	presenting	rupture
cord prolapse	forewaters	presentation	twin

Table 11.3

	Indications to perform vaginal examination
a.	To assess _____ or _____ in labour.
b.	To confirm the _____ of the _____
c.	To make a positive identification of _____
d.	To determine whether the (head) is _____ (in case of doubt).
e.	To ascertain whether the _____ have _____ , or to _____ them artificially.
f.	To exclude _____ after _____ of the _____ especially if there is an _____ part or the _____ rate changes.
g.	In multiple pregnancy: To confirm the _____ of the fetus and _____ of the second _____ and, if necessary, in order to _____ the second _____ sac.

5. Table 11.4 relates to the possible findings a midwife can obtain from performing a vaginal examination. Complete the table by providing the full response or inserting the missing word(s) to complete the statements. Refer to textbook if required.

Table 11.4

Findings	Detail possible findings on vaginal examination
a. Observations noted:	i. Labia for any sign of _____ _____. ii. Perineum for any _____ _____. iii. Vaginal orifice: _____. iv. Other observation (if present): _____ _____.
b. Maternal	i. Rectum: _____. ii. (In multiparous women): _____.
c. Cervix	_____ and _____. _____ of the _____ canal, _____ of cervix and _____ to the presenting part.
d. Membranes (with description)	i. _____ or _____. ii. _____ _____.
e. Presenting part (96% vertex presents)	i. _____ – estimation in relationship to maternal _____ noting the distance _____ or _____ the _____. ii. The presence of _____ or _____.
f. Position and flexion	The position of the _____ as defined by the _____ including _____ (using any _____ and _____ located).
g. Rotation	Noting changes in the _____ of the fetus from a previous assessment.

Fetal heart rate

 Completion

6. Table 11.5 provides definitions for changes in fetal heart rate. Complete the definitions by inserting the words and numerical values from the list provided (options may be used more than once).

rise	deceleration	baseline	5	15
drop	vary		3	1

Table 11.5

Category	Definition
a. Acceleration	This is a brief _____ in the fetal heart rate of at least _____ beats, for at least _____ s.
b. Deceleration	This is a _____ in the fetal heart rate from the _____ of _____ beats for >_____ s but <_____ min.
c. Bradycardia	This is a _____ of the fetal heart rate lasting longer than _____ min.
d. Baseline rate	Baseline rate should _____ by at least ____ beats over a period of ____ min.

7. Table 11.6 presents the classification of fetal heart rate trace features (classified by NICE 2007). Complete the missing sections of the table by inserting the correct word/numerical values from the extended list provided (options may be used more than once).

acceleration	deceleration	present	typical	5	40	90	110	180
atypical	late	prolonged	variable	10	50	100	160	
early	none	sinusoidal	3	30	60	109	161	

Table 11.6

	Feature	Baseline (bpm)	Variability (bpm)	Decelerations	Accelerations
	a. Reassuring	_____–_____	≥5	_____	_____
	b. Non-reassuring	_____–_____ _____–_____	<5 for _____–_____ minutes	_____ variable decelerations with over 50% of contractions, occurring for over _____ minutes. Single _____ deceleration for up to _____ minutes.	The absence of accelerations with an otherwise normal CTG are of uncertain significance
E.F.M	c. Abnormal	<_____ >_____ _____ pattern for ≤_____ minutes	<5 for _____ minutes	Either _____ variable decelerations with over 50% of contractions or _____ decelerations, both for over _____ minutes. Single _____ deceleration for more than ____ minutes.	

8. Table 11.7 presents the definition of normal, suspicious and pathological fetal heart rate (FHR) traces (NICE 2007). Complete the definitions for each category.

Table 11.7

Category	Definition
a. Normal	A FHR trace in which _____ _____
b. Suspicious	A FHR trace with _____ _____ _____
c. Pathological	A FHR trace with _____ _____ _____

Physiological response to pain and pain pathways

 Completion

9. Complete the following paragraph about the physiological response to pain by removing the incorrect word(s) so that it reads correctly.

Pain of labour is associated with an **increased/decreased** respiratory rate. This may cause a **decrease/increase** in $PaCO_2$ level with a corresponding **increase/decrease** in pH. The fetus is then affected and a subsequent **rise/drop** in the fetal $PaCO_2$ ensues. This may be suspected by the presence of **late/early** decelerations on the CTG. The acid–base equilibrium of the system may be altered by **hyper/hypo**ventilation. **Acidosis/alkalosis** may then affect the diffusion of **oxygen/carbon dioxide** across the placenta leading to a degree of fetal hypoxia.

Cardiac output **increases/decreases** by **20%/50%** in first stage and **20/50%** in second stage of labour. Pain apprehension and fear may cause a **sympathetic/non-sympathetic** response thereby producing more of an **increase/decrease** in cardiac output.

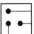 **Labelling**

10. Figure 11.2 describes the sensory pathway showing the structures involved in the appreciation of pain. Label the figure using the list of structures and tissues provided.

Anterior aspect of spinal cord

Nerve cells in medulla oblongata

Sensory decussation

2nd neuron

Basal ganglia

Pons Varolii

Sensory nerve ending in skin receptor

3rd neuron

Cerebral cortex

Posterior (or dorsal) horn contains substantia gelatinosa

Thalamus

Internal capsule

Posterior root ganglion

1st neuron

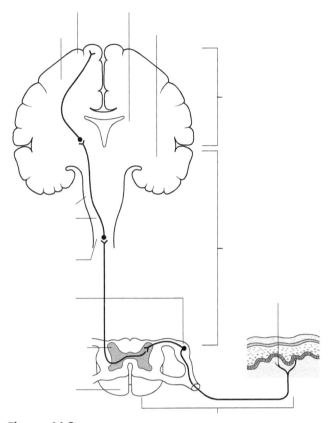

Figure 11.2

  Colouring and labelling

11. Figure 11.3 presents pain pathways showing the site at which pain may be intercepted by local anaesthetic techniques. Using the lists provided, colour and label the figure as detailed.

Colour and label

Site for caudal epidural block

Site for epidural and spinal blocks

Site for paracervical block

Site for pudendal block

Label

Lumbar vertebrae 1–5

Pudendal nerve

Sacral vertebrae

Thoracic vertebrae 11 and 12

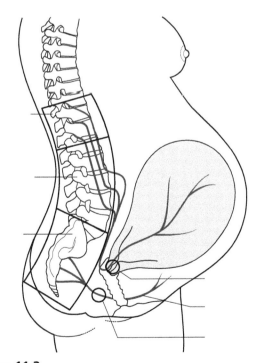

Figure 11.3

12. Figure 11.4 shows a sagittal section of the lumbar spine with Tuohy needle in position.

Colour and label

Spinal process
Epidural space
Inter- and supraspinous ligaments
Ligamentum flavum
Spinal cord
Intervertebral discs

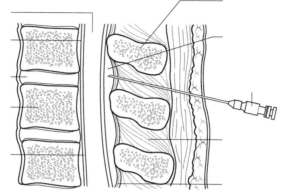

Label

Dura mater
Body of vertebra
Subarachnoid space

Figure 11.4

 True/false

13. Complete Table 11.8 by deciding if the statements are true or false by ticking the appropriate column.

Table 11.8

	Statements	True	False
a.	The retraction ring continues to rise once the cervix is fully dilated and the fetus leaves the uterus.		
b.	The presenting part is defined as the part of the fetus lying over the uterine os during labour.		
c.	In multiparous women a perceptible cervical canal may remain.		
d.	In the rare event of a sacculated retroverted gravid uterus the cervix may be located in an extreme posterior position.		
e.	Oestrogen stimulates the placenta to release prostaglandins that induce a production of enzymes that soften the cervix by digesting the collagen.		
f.	High levels of oestrogen cause uterine muscle fibres to display oxytocic receptors and form gap junctions with each other.		
g.	Endorphins are found in the: limbic system, hypothalamus and reticular formation.		
h.	Levels of maternal oestrogen rise sharply during the last weeks of pregnancy resulting in promoting the effects of progesterone.		
i.	Nitrous oxide (N_2O) acts by limiting the neuronal and synaptic transmission within the CNS.		

? **Multiple choice questions (MCQs)**

14. The incidence of pre-labour rupture of membranes (PROM) at term is:

a. 2–6%   b. 8–10%   c. 0–14%   d. 15–20%

15. The process of synthesizing glucose from non-carbohydrate sources is termed:

a. Glycogenesis

b. Glycogenolysis

c. Gluconeogenesis

d. None of the above

16. Mendelson's syndrome is:

a. A chemical pneumonitis caused by the inhalation of gastric contents

b. Excessive production of gastric acid during labour

c. Reduction in gastrointestinal activity during pregnancy

d. An increase in blood pressure during labour

17. Sensory receptors that respond to pain are called:

    a. Proprioreceptors

    b. Baroreceptors

    c. Nociceptors

    d. Somatic receptors

18. The gate-control theory declares that:

    a. A neural or spinal gating mechanism occurs in the substantia gelatinosa of the dorsal horns of the spinal cord

    b. A neural or spinal gating mechanism occurs in the substantia gelatinosa of the anterior horns of the spinal cord

    c. It is the size of the gate that determines whether or not the nerve impulses travel freely to the medulla and thalamus

    d. Nerve impulses received by the receptors for pain are unaffected by the gating mechanism

19. Transcutaneous electrical nerve stimulation:

    a. Stimulates the production of natural endorphins and enkephalins

    b. Stimulates low threshold efferent fibres leading to inhibition of nerve fibres

    c. The two electrodes situated between S1 and S4 provide pain control mainly during first stage of labour

    d. All of the above

    e. None of the above

20. Periods of 'fetal sleep' noted on CTG commonly last for:

    a. 3–5 min

    b. 5–7 min

    c. 10–15 min

    d. 20–30 min

SECOND STAGE OF LABOUR

 Definitions

21. Complete Table 11.9 and using your own words, define the second stage of labour.

Table 11.9

Stage	Definition
Second stage	The second stage begins _____. In physiological labour the woman usually feels the _____ to _____ the fetus. It is complete when the _____.

Definitions and completion

22. Table 11.10 presents definitions related to labour. Complete this table by providing the correct missing word(s) from the list provided (options may be used more than once).

abdominal	forward	coccyx	presenting	buttocks
applied	dome	diaphragm	pigmented	powers
curve	fundal contraction	sacrum	cleft	push
compulsive	lower	upper pole	posterior	presenting part
contraction	anal cleft	long axis	occiput	pelvic floor
expulsion	involuntary	nerve	pressure	

Table 11.10

	Definitions	
a.	Fetal axis pressure	This occurs during _____ when the uterus rises _____ and the force of the _____ is transmitted to the _____ of the fetus, down the _____ of the fetus and _____ by the _____ part to the cervix.
b.	'Purple line'	This is a _____ mark in the _____ of the _____ which creeps up the _____ as labour progresses. It is also called the '_____ line'.
c.	Rhomboid of Michaelis	This presents as a _____ shaped _____ in the _____ back, and is held to indicate the _____ displacement of the _____ and _____ as the fetal _____ moves into the maternal _____.
d.	'Ferguson's reflex'	This phenomenon occurs when _____ from the _____ stimulates _____ receptors in the _____. The woman experiences the need to _____ and this becomes increasingly, _____, overwhelming and _____. Maternal response is to employ secondary _____ of _____ by contracting her _____ muscles and _____.

 Completion

23. The following statements relate to the soft tissue displacement during second stage. Complete the following statements to read correctly by inserting the missing words from the list provided.

| levator ani muscles | rectum | sacral curve |
| bladder | perineal body | urethra |

a. Anteriorly, the _____ is pushed upwards into the abdomen.

b. The _____ is stretched and thins out so that the lumen is reduced.

c. Posteriorly, the _____ becomes flattened into the _____.

d. The _____ dilate, thin out and are displaced laterally.

e. The _____ is flattened, stretched and thinned.

24. List three favourable positions to promote descent and progress in labour.

_____ _____ _____

25. List four physiological factors that make these positions more favourable for second stage labour.

_____

_____

_____

_____

Mechanisms of labour

The following activities relate to the mechanism of labour which is a collective term for the movements involved as the fetus descends through the birth canal. Knowledge and recognition of normal mechanism enables the midwife to anticipate the next steps in the process of descent.

✎ Completion

26. Complete the following principles common to all mechanisms.

a.   _____ takes place.

b.   Whichever part leads and first meets the _____ of the pelvic floor will

_____ forward until it comes under the _____.

c.   Whatever emerges from the _____ will pivot around the _____.

Mechanisms are described using a systematic stem with relevant information inserted for each labour. The following mechanism relates to the most common – vertex presentation with either a right or left occipitoanterior position.

27. Complete the following statements by inserting the missing words.

a.   The lie is _____

b.   The presentation is _____

c.   The position is right or left _____

d.   The attitude is one of _____

e.   The _____ is the occiput

f.   The presenting part is the _____ part of the _____

_____.

Matching and labelling

The following activities relate to the main movements as the fetus descends through the birth canal. A list of movements is provided.

28. Complete the flow diagram of the sequence of events inserting the movements from the list provided.

Descent   Flexion   Internal rotation of the shoulders   Restitution

Extension of the head   Internal rotation of the head   Lateral flexion

_____ → _____ →

_____ → _____

_____ → _____ → _____

_____ → _____.

Matching

29. Complete the following statements in Table 11.11 by matching the statement to the movement referred to in the list previously provided in Question 28. Movements from the list may be used more than once.

Table 11.11

	Statement	Movement
a.	This increases throughout labour and relates to the fetal spine being attached nearer to the posterior skull.	
b.	The twist in the neck is now corrected by a slight untwisting movement.	
c.	In multigravid women this may not occur until labour actually begins.	
d.	Resistance of the pelvic floor is an important determinant in bringing this movement about.	
e.	The occiput slips beneath the sub-pubic arch and crowning occurs when the head no longer recedes between contractions.	
f.	The slope of the pelvic floor determines the direction of this movement.	
g.	Pressure exerted down the fetal axis will be more forcibly transmitted to the occiput than the sinciput.	
h.	During this movement, the fetal head pivots on the suboccipital region around the pubic bone.	
i.	The remainder of the body is born as the spine bends sideways through the curved birth canal.	
j.	The sinciput, face, and chin are released and sweep the perineum.	
k.	In a well-flexed vertex presentation the occiput leads and rotates anteriorly 1/8th circle causing a slight twist in the neck.	
l.	The occiput moves 1/8th of a circle towards the side of the head from which it started.	
m.	The anterior shoulder is the first to reach the levator ani muscle and rotates anteriorly to lie under the symphysis pubis.	

Perineal trauma

 Completion

30. Table 11.12 relates to classification of degrees of spontaneous tears. Complete the table by inserting the missing word(s) from the list provided. Note that a few words may be used more than once.

anal sphincter	fourchette	perineal	superficial
complete	internal	pubococcygeus	transverse
external	partial	rectal mucosa	

Table 11.12

	Tear	Structures
a.	1-degree	Involves _____ only.
b.	2-degree	Involves the _____ and the _____ _____ muscles, namely the _____ _____ muscles and in some cases the _____.
c.	3-degree	Comprises a _____ or _____ disruption of the _____ _____ muscles, which may involve either or both _____ and _____ _____ muscles.
d.	4-degree	Involves a disruption of the _____ muscles with a breach of the _____ _____.

31. Define the term 'episiotomy': An episiotomy is an _____

_____

_____

32. Name the two main directions of episiotomy: a. _____

b. _____.

Miscellaneous

 True/false

33. Complete the following statements in Table 11.13 by deciding if they are true or false by ticking the appropriate column.

Table 11.13

	Statement	True	False
a.	Caput succedaneum does not usually protrude through the cervix prior to full dilatation of the os.		
b.	External rotation of the head occurs at the same time as internal rotation of the shoulders.		
c.	If flexion is maintained during descent then it will be the suboccipitobregmatic diameter that distends the vaginal orifice.		
d.	The widest diameter of the pelvic brim is the transverse.		
e.	Left lateral position may aid fetal rotation.		
f.	Epidural analgesia causes relaxation of the pelvic floor and delays internal rotation of the head.		
g.	In the case of occipitoposterior positions women report the 'all fours position' to be beneficial in reducing backache.		

Multiple choice questions (MCQs)

34. Breath-holding and attempting to exhale against closed airways is called:

    a. McRobert's manoeuvre

    b. Valsalva manoeuvre

    c. Rubin manoeuvre

    d. Ferguson's reflex

35. In the semi-recumbent or supporting sitting position:

    a. The woman's weight is on her sacrum

    b. The coccyx is directed posteriorly

    c. The pelvic outlet is increased

    d. All of the above

    e. None of the above

36. The time taken for Lidocaine (local anaesthetic) to take effect is:

    a. <1 minute

    b. Between 1 and 2 minutes

    c. Between 3 and 4 minutes

    d. >4 minutes

37. When the membranes remain intact this:

    a. Optimizes the oxygen supply to the fetus

    b. Helps prevent intrauterine and fetal infection

    c. Ensures the general fluid pressure is equalized throughout the uterus and over the fetal body

    d. All of the above

    e. None of the above

Reference

NICE (2007) Intrapartum Care Guideline. [Online] Available at: http://www.nice.org.uk/CG055fullguideline [Accessed 24 April 2012].

CHAPTER

12 Third stage of labour

This chapter focuses on the normal physiological mechanisms of placental separation and descent together with factors that facilitate haemostasis and primary postpartum haemorrhage. This midwife has a key role to play in providing safe and effective care and to anticipate, recognize and act promptly and competently when haemorrhage occurs. The activities will test your knowledge in these areas.

 Definition

1. Complete the following activity in Table 12.1 relating to third stage by providing a detailed definition and inserting the correct numerical values.

Table 12.1

	Definition
a. Third stage	This is the period from the _____ _____ _____
b. Duration	Active management of the third stage of labour is diagnosed as prolonged if not completed within _____ minutes of the birth of the baby (NICE 2007). Physiological management of the third stage of labour is diagnosed as prolonged if not completed within _____ minutes of the birth of the baby (NICE 2007).

Physiology of third stage

The following activities relate to the factors involved in separation and expulsion of the placental and membranes, i.e mechanical and haemostatic factors. It is difficult to separate these two factors completely as they take place simultaneously during the process.

 Completion

2. Flow diagram 12.1 details the mechanical factors involved in the separation of the placenta. Complete the sections by inserting the missing word(s) to read correctly from the list provided. A few word(s) may be used more than once and you will be required to insert the numerical value required.

accelerate	decidua basalis	membranes	retraction
attachment	diminished	non-elastic	spongy
compressed	distended	placental	tortuous
congested	forcing	placental site	vagina
contracts	intervillous spaces	oblique	
detach	lower uterine segment	reduces	

Flow diagram 12.1:

a. During second stage, the uterine cavity progressively empties, enabling the _____

    process to _____. At the beginning of third stage, the _____

    has already _____ in area by about _____%.

    ↓

b. As this occurs, the placenta becomes _____ and the blood in the _____

    _____ is forced back into the _____ layer of the _____.

    _____ of the _____ uterine muscle fibres exerts pressure on

    the blood vessels so that blood does not drain back into the maternal system. The vessels during this process

    are termed '_____' as they become tense and _____ with blood.

    ↓

c. With the next contraction, the _____ veins burst and a small amount of blood seeps

    in between the septa of the _____ layer and the _____

    surface, stripping it from its _____. As the surface for attachment

    _____, the relatively _____ placenta begins to

    _____ from the uterine wall.

    ↓

d. Once separation has occurred, the uterus _____ strongly, _____ placenta

    and _____ to fall into the _____ and finally into the

    _____.

Placental separation

  Colouring and completion

3. Figure 12.1 shows the mechanism of placental separation. Consider the previous activity and complete as
   noted.

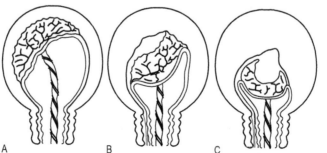

Colour

uterine wall
fetal surface of placenta
maternal surface of placenta

A   B   C

Figure 12.1

Complete the following:

a. Figure 12.1 (A) shows _____

b. Figure 12.1 (B) shows _____

c. Figure 12.1 (C) shows _____

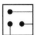 **Colouring, labelling and completion**

4. These activities relate to the two methods of expulsion of the placenta detailed in Table 12.2 and shown in Figure 12.2. Colour, label and complete the following related activities as noted.

  Colour

a. Colour the areas listed on Figure 12.2.

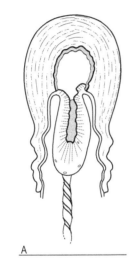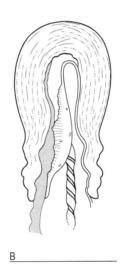

Fetal surface
Maternal surface
Myometrium
Bleeding from site

A _____   B _____

Figure 12.2A & B

  Label

b. Identify and label method of expulsion of placenta (A) and (B) on Figure 12.2.

c. Complete Table 12.2 by providing/removing the information as requested for the two methods of placental separation.

Table 12.2

	Method (A)	Method (B)
a. Label this method.	_____	_____
b. Where does separation begin?	_____	_____
c. Is a retroplacental clot involved?	Yes/no	Yes/no
d. Which surface appears first?	_____	_____
e. Difference in duration between methods?	Shorter/longer	Shorter/longer
fi. Difference in blood loss between methods?	More/less	More/less
g. Detail possible visible differences on examination?	_____ _____ _____	_____ _____ _____

Haemostasis and the role in placental separation

 Completion

5. The following paragraphs relate to haemostasis and the role it has in placental separation. Complete the following paragraphs by removing the incorrect word(s) so that it reads correctly.

The normal volume of blood flow through a healthy placental site is **500–800/300–500** mL/min. Serious haemorrhage would occur at the time of placental separation if blood flow was not arrested within **seconds/ minutes**. An interplay of the following three factors to control bleeding within the normal physiological processes is essential during this stage:

a. The **tortuous/relaxed** blood vessels **intertwine through/run adjacent to** the **oblique/circular** uterine muscle fibres. **Retraction/relaxation** of the **oblique/longitudinal** uterine muscle fibres in the **upper/lower** uterine segment results in **thinning/thickening** of the muscles. This exerts pressure on the torn vessels, acting as clamps so securing a ligature action.

b. Presence of **vigorous/gentle** uterine contraction following separation brings the **placenta/uterine** walls into apposition so that **further/less** pressure is exerted on the umbilical **cord/placental site**.

c. Haemostasis is achieved by a transitory **deactivation/activation** of the coagulation and fibrinolytic systems during, and immediately following, placental separation. This protective response is especially **dormant/active** at the placental site so that clot formation in the **intact/torn** vessels is **diminished/ intensified**. Following separation, the placental site is **gradually/rapidly** covered by a **platelet/fibrin** mesh utilizing **5–10%/15–25%** of circulating **platelets/fibrinogen**.

Uterotonic drugs

 Matching

6. Consider each statement in Table 12.3 relating to common uterotonic drugs used during the third stage. Complete the table by choosing the correct drug each statement refers to by ticking the appropriate column.

Table 12.3

	Statement	Ergometrine	Oxytocin
a.	This drug is the synthetic form of a hormone (to stimulate smooth muscle contraction) produced in the posterior pituitary gland.		
b.	If ergometrine and oxytocin are combined then 1 mL ampoule will contain 5 IU of this drug.		
c.	If ergometrine and oxytocin are combined then 1 mL ampoule will contain 0.5 mg of this drug.		
d.	If administered intramuscularly then this drug will act within 2.5 minutes.		
e.	If this drug is administered as an IV bolus then it should be administered slowly due to profound and potentially fatal hypotensive side-effects.		
f.	If administered intramuscularly then this drug will act within 6–7 minutes.		
g.	This drug is contraindicated if there is a history of hypertensive or cardiac disease.		

Short answers

7. Complete the following statements:

a. The commonly used brand name of oxytocin is _____.

b. The commonly used brand name of the combined drug ergometrine and oxytocin is

_____.

c. The combined action of ergometrine and oxytocin results in a _____

_____

_____

d. At birth, the timing of administration of a uterotonic drug is usually as the _____

_____

e. The side-effects of the combined drug (ergometrine and oxytocin) include _____

_____.

8. Complete the following activities related to the management of third stage (i.e. uterotonic drugs, the umbilical cord, delivery of the placenta and membranes).

a. Active management policy usually includes the following three key processes:

i. _____

ii. _____

_____

iii. _____

b. Expectant or physiological management usually involves the following processes:

i. _____

ii. _____

iii. _____

9. List the signs that indicate the placenta has separated and descent has occurred.

_____

_____

_____

True/false

10. Consider the statements in Table 12.4. Decide if they are true or false and complete the table by ticking the correct column.

Table 12.4

	Statement	True	False
a.	The placenta <u>always</u> shears off the uterine wall during the final contraction.		
b.	It is the absence of oblique fibres in the lower uterine segment that explains the greatly increased blood loss usually accompanying placental separation in placenta praevia.		
c.	The unique characteristic of uterine muscle lies in its power of retraction.		
d.	Uterotonic drugs are always administered after the birth of the baby and prior to placental delivery.		
e.	Prostaglandins are never recommended for use in third stage management.		
f.	In CTT, it is vital to provide counter-traction to prevent inversion of the uterus.		
g.	Due to side effects, <u>only</u> 1 dose of ergometrine (0.5 mg) should be routinely administered.		
h.	In situations of haemorrhage due to hypotonic uterine action then intravenous ergometrine is used as it secures a rapid contraction in 45 seconds.		

Complications of the third stage

 Completion

11. Complete the following definitions/statements in Table 12.5 referring to the textbook as required.

Table 12.5

		Definition
a.	Primary postpartum haemorrhage (PPH)	This relates to _____ bleeding from the _____ _____
b.	Blood loss	Irrespective of maternal condition, blood loss reaching _____ mL must be treated as a PPH.
c.	Secondary postpartum haemorrhage	This relates to any _____ or _____ bleeding from the _____ occurring between _____ hours and _____ weeks postnatally.

12. List the four reasons why a PPH might occur:

_____   _____

_____   _____

Atonic uterus

13. Complete the following activities relating to atonic uterus. A word list is provided as prompts for activities 13 a, b (i–iii). You can refer to the textbook for the remainder of the activities.

abruption	effective	exhaustion	precipitate	prolonged
compress	Couvelaire	muscle	polyhydramnios	praevia
contract	living ligature	myometrium	placental site	retract
control	lower segment	multiple pregnancy	oblique	thinner

a. Complete the following paragraph by inserting the missing words so that it reads correctly.

An atonic uterus relates to the failure of the _____ at the _____

to _____ and _____ and to _____ torn blood vessels and

_____ blood loss by a _____ action.

b. Complete Table 12.6 relating to the causes of atonic uterine action.

Table 12.6

	List the possible causes relating to:
i. Pregnancy related	_____ or _____ causing overdistension of the uterine muscle.
ii. Conditions affecting the placenta	Placenta _____ as it partly or wholly lies in the _____ _____ where the _____ muscle layer contains few _____ fibres resulting in poor control of bleeding. Placenta _____ as blood may have seeped between the _____ fibres interfering with _____ muscle action. A severe case results in a _____ uterus.
iii. Labour	_____ labour and _____ labour resulting in uterine inertia resulting from maternal _____ / sluggishness.
iv. Placental separation	
v. Maternal reasons	_____ may be a mechanical reason that interferes with uterine action.
vi. Other	_____ which may cause uterine _____ , e.g. halothane.

Primary postpartum haemorrhage

✎ Completion

14. List four other factors that increase the possibility of, although do not directly cause PPH.

_____   _____

_____   _____

It is vital that students know the three basic principles of care applied immediately upon observing excessive bleeding. These are: 1) call for help; 2) stop the bleeding and 3) resuscitate the mother.

Completion

15. Figure 12.3 provides a detailed flow of action to be taken in a primary PPH. Review the flow diagram and insert the missing words so that the flow reads correctly.

Apply pressure, repair the wound	In lower uterine segment	Placenta delivered
Controlled cord traction	IV infusion syntocinon 40 u/L	Rub up a contraction
Empty the uterus	Lift the legs	Separated
Ergometrine 0.5 mg IV	Lower genital tract injury	Uterus firmly contracted
Give an oxytocic	Measures fail to arrest bleeding	

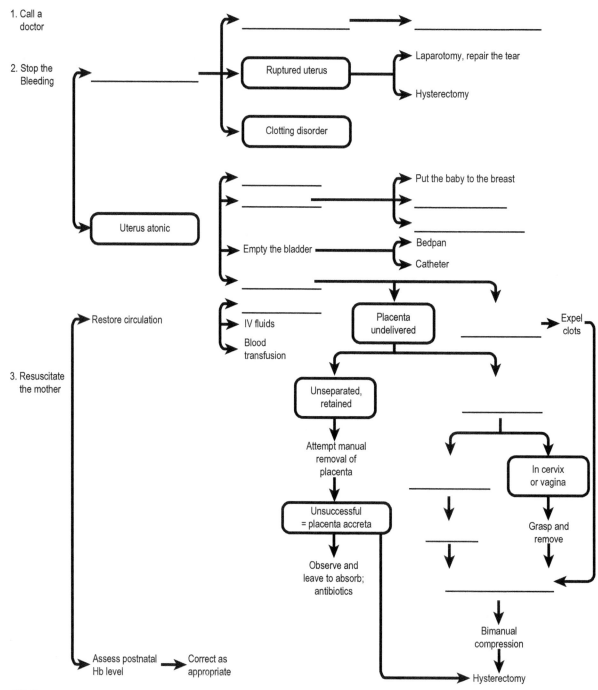

Figure 12.3

Bimanual compression

16. Bimanual compression of the uterus may be required to apply pressure to the placental site if bleeding continues. Complete the following paragraph by removing the incorrect word(s) so that it reads correctly.

The fingers of one hand are inserted into the vagina like a **fist/cone**; the hand is formed into a **cone/fist** and placed into the **posterior/anterior** vaginal **fornix/orifice**, the **wrist/elbow** resting on the bed. The other hand is placed behind the uterus **vaginally/abdominally**, the fingers pointing **away from/towards** the cervix. The **cervix/uterus** is brought **backwards/forwards** and compressed between the **back/palm** of the hand positioned **anteriorly/abdominally** and the **cone/fist** in the vagina.

 ## True/false

17. Consider the following statements in Table 12.7. Decide if the statements are true or false and complete the table by ticking the appropriate column.

Table 12.7

	Statement	True	False
a.	The main symptom of haematoma formation is increasingly severe maternal pain.		
b.	One benefit of breastfeeding immediately following birth is the reflex release of prolactin from the posterior pituitary gland which stimulates the uterus to contract.		
c.	Haematoma formation only occurs in the perineum and lower vagina.		
d.	On palpation, an enlarged uterus filling with blood or blood clots feels soft and distended and lacking tone. The uterus is described as being 'boggy'.		
e.	In placenta accreta, the placenta remains morbidly adherent to the uterine wall.		
f.	Cord blood sampling is usually taken when atypical maternal antibodies have been found during antenatal screening test.		

Reference

NICE (2007) Intrapartum Care Guideline. [Online] Available at: http://www.nice.org.uk/CG055fullguideline [Accessed 24 April 2012].

13 Complicated labour and birth

This chapter focuses on complicated labour and births. These situations including malpositions and malpresentations of the fetus can be challenging for the midwife who has a key role in the recognition and diagnosis during pregnancy and labour. The activities will test your knowledge in the variety of related areas of practice.

Prolonged pregnancy and induction of labour

✎ Completion

1. Complete the following statements by inserting the correct numerical value.

   a. The legal definition of the age of fetal viability in the UK is _____ weeks.

   b. Women with uncomplicated pregnancies should usually be offered induction of labour between _____

   and _____ weeks to avoid the risks of prolonged pregnancy (NICE 2008).

   c. In relation to the Bishop's score, a score of _____ or above equates with a ripe cervix.

   d. In precipitate labour, the uterus is over-efficient and the time (hour(s)) from the onset of labour to birth is

   ___ hour(s) or less.

True/false

2. Consider the following statements in Table 13.1. Complete the table by deciding if the statements are correct by ticking the appropriate column.

Table 13.1

	Statement	True	False
a.	Prolonged pregnancy refers to a specific gestation and does not relate to the fetus or neonate.		
b.	Prostaglandins are naturally occurring female hormones present in tissues throughout the body.		
c.	Pre-labour rupture of membranes is a maternal indication for IOL.		
d.	NICE (2008) recommend sweeping of the membranes prior to formal induction procedures at 40+ weeks or earlier where there are complications.		
e.	Prostaglandin E2 placed in the posterior fornix of the vagina is absorbed by the epithelium of the vagina and cervix leading to relaxation and dilatation of the muscle of the cervix.		
f.	As an alternative approach to initiating labour, stimulation of the nipple/breast does not appear to cause the release of endogenous oxytocin.		
g.	Dystocia is the term used for difficult or slow labour and includes failure to progress and prolonged labour.		
h.	As the uterus continues to contract and retract in obstructed labour, the upper segment becomes progressively thinner and the lower segment becomes increasingly thicker.		

Completion

3. Table 13.2 show the modified Bishop's score. Complete the table by inserting the missing words and numerical values. Refer to textbook if required.

Table 13.2

Inducibility features	0	1	2	3
_____ of the cervix (cm)	<1	__-__	__-__	>__
Consistency of the _____	_____	_____	Med	_____
Cervical canal _____ (cm)	>__	__-__	__-__	<1
_____ of the cervix	_____	Mid	_____	N/A
Station of _____ (cm above or below ischial spines)	____	____	__,__	+1, +2

Malpositions of the occiput

 True/false

4. Consider the statements in Table 13.3 related to occipitoposterior position. Decide if they are true or false and complete the table by ticking the correct column.

Table 13.3

	Statement	True	False
a.	The fetal head is deflexed and smaller diameters of the fetal skull may present.		
b.	The oval shape of the anthropoid pelvis favours a direct occipitoposterior position.		
c.	On inspection, there is a saucer-shaped depression at or just below the umbilicus.		
d.	On palpation, the occiput and sinciput can be located on the same level.		
e.	On auscultation, the fetal heart may be heard more easily at the flank on the same side as the back.		
f.	The membranes tend to rupture spontaneously at an early stage of labour.		
g.	On vaginal examination, locating the anterior fontanelle in the anterior part of the pelvis is diagnostic.		
h.	The woman does not usually experience backache during labour.		

 Labelling and completion

5. The following activities relate to the diameters and dimensions of a deflexed head.

    a. Figure 13.1 shows the engaging diameter of a deflexed head. Label the diameter and identify the length (cm).

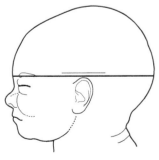

Figure 13.1 Engaging diameter of a deflexed head.

b. Figure 13.2 shows the presenting dimensions
   of a deflexed head. Label the diameters,
   identifying the length (cm) and insert the
   numerical value (cm) of the circumference.

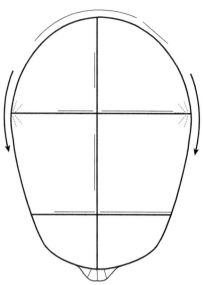

Figure 13.2 Presenting dimensions of a deflexed head.

 Completion

There are two possible outcomes for occipitoposterior positions of the occiput, i.e. long rotation and short
rotation. The following activities relate to the mechanism of labour in right occipitoposterior position (Figures
13.3–13.6).

6. Complete Table 13.4 by inserting the correct word(s) to complete the mechanism of right occipitoposterior
position (long rotation).

Table 13.4

	Mechanism of right occipitoposterior position (long rotation)
a.	The lie is _____.
b.	The attitude of the head is _____.
c.	The presentation is _____.
d.	The position is _____.
e.	The _____ is the occiput.
f.	The presenting part is the _____.
g.	The _____ diameter (_____ cm) lies in the right _____ diameter of the pelvic brim. The occiput points to the right sacroiliac joint and the sinciput to the left _____ _____.

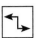 ## Matching and completion

7. Review the following Figures 13.3–13.6 showing the mechanisms of labour in right occipitoposterior position. Complete the activities in Tables 13.5 A and B in relation to flexion, descent and rotation movements by inserting the missing information from the list provided.

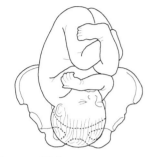 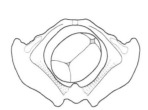

Figure 13.3

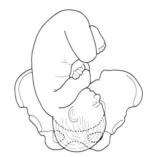 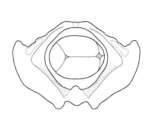

Figure 13.4

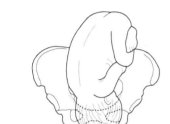 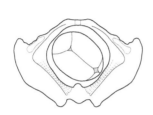

Figure 13.5

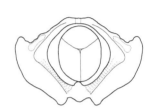

Figure 13.6

anterior	descent	posterior	occipitoanterior	1/8th
crowning	extension	oblique	symphysis pubis	2/8th
internal	flexion	occiput	sagittal	3/8th
external	forwards	twist	transverse	right
lateral flexion	restitution	perineum	sinciput	

Table 13.5A

	Mechanism	Description
a.	Descent and flexion Figure 13.3	_____ takes place with increasing _____. _____ suture lies in the right _____ diameter of the pelvis. The _____ becomes the leading part.
b.	Internal rotation of the head (b, c & d) Figure 13.4	The _____ and shoulders have rotated ____ th(s) of a circle _____. _____ suture lies in the _____ diameter of the pelvis.
c	Figure 13.5	The _____ and shoulders have rotated ____ th(s) of a circle _____. _____ suture now lies in the left _____ diameter of the pelvis. The position is right _____.
d.	Figure 13.6	The _____ has rotated _____th(s) of a circle _____ to lie under the _____. There is a _____ in the neck. _____ suture lies in the _____ diameter of the pelvis.

Continued →

The information in this table continues on from the Table 13.5A (a–d). Complete the table by inserting the missing words/values (e–j) for the mechanism of right OP position long rotation.

Table 13.5B

	Mechanism	Description
e.	_____	The occiput escapes under the symphysis pubis.
f.	_____	The _____, face, and chin sweep the _____ and the head is born by a movement of _____.
g.	_____	The occiput turns ____ th(s) of a circle to the _____ and the head realigns with the shoulders.
h.	_____ rotation of the shoulders	The shoulders enter the pelvis in the right oblique diameter; the _____ shoulder reaches the pelvic floor first and rotates ____ th(s) of a circle to lie under the symphysis pubis.
i.	_____ rotation of the head	At the same time the _____ turns a further ____ th(s) of a circle to the _____.
j.	_____ _____	The _____ shoulder escapes under the symphysis pubis, the _____ shoulder sweeps the perineum and the body is born by _____ _____.

8. Figure 13.7 shows the 'persistent occipitoposterior position' <u>before</u> rotation of the occiput and Figure 13.8 shows 'persistent occipitoposterior position <u>after</u> short rotation. Consider these figures and complete the following paragraph by either removing the incorrect word or inserting the correct word so that it reads correctly.

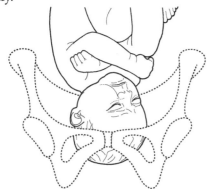

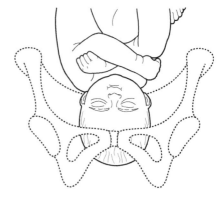

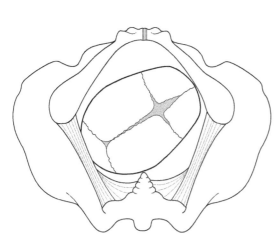

Figure 13.7

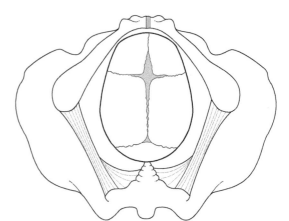

Figure 13.8

The position in Figure 13.7 is **right/left** occipitoposterior. The _____ fails to rotate forwards in this situation. Instead the **occiput/sinciput** reaches the pelvic floor first and rotates **backwards/forwards**. The **occiput/sinciput** goes into the hollow of the sacrum. The position in Figure 13.8 is _____ _____. The baby is born facing the _____. This is termed a '_____ to _____' birth.

Fetal malpresentations

 Matching

9. Complete the following activity by matching the statements in Table 13.6 to the correct presentation (i.e. face, brow or breech presentations).

Table 13.6

	Statement	Presentation
a.	This may result in obstructed labour with a caesarean section being the probable outcome.	
b.	Anencephaly can be a fetal cause.	
c.	The denominator is the sacrum.	Breech
d.	The presenting diameter is the mentovertical.	
e.	The incidence is about ≤1:500.	
f.	Vaginal birth is rare.	
g.	The incidence at term is approximately 3%.	
h.	The denominator is the mentum.	
i.	The incidence is approximately 1:1000 deliveries.	
j.	The fetal heart heard clearly above the umbilicus when engagement has not yet occurred.	

 Labelling and completion

10. Figure 13.9 shows the diameters involved in the delivery of face presentation. Complete the following activity on Figure 13.9.

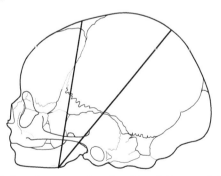

Figure 13.9 Diameters involved in delivery of face presentation.

Label (name and length)

Engaging diameter
Diameter that sweeps the perineum

Completion

11. Complete the missing word(s) in Table 13.7.

Table 13.7

	Mechanism of a left mentoanterior position
a.	The lie is _____ .
b.	The attitude is one of _____ of the _____ .
c.	The presentation is _____ .
d.	The position is _____ .
e.	The denominator is the _____ .
f.	The presenting part is the _____ .

 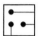 **Colouring and labelling**

12. Figure 13.10 shows the diameter that lies at the back of the pelvic brim in a brow presentation. The length of this diameter exceeds all diameters in an average-sized pelvis.

Label

Name this diameter and identify the length (cm).

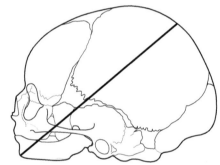

Figure 13.10 Brow presentation.

13. After birth, the shape of the baby's head as a result of moulding gives an indication of the presentation during labour. The following activities relate to the types of moulding. For activities a, b, c, d you are required to name the diameter(s), provide the length in cm and colour the dashed or dotted line you will insert to indicate moulding (where relevant).

   a. Figure 13.11 shows the type of moulding in a vertex presentation.

Label

The two most common diameters and identify the length (cm) in a vertex presentation.

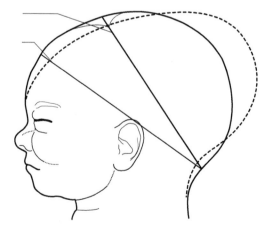

Figure 13.11 Type of moulding in a vertex presentation.

Colour and label (b–d)

b. Figure 13.12 shows the head in a persistent occipitoposterior position. Label the diameter, identify the length (cm) and colour in a dashed line to show the direction of moulding.

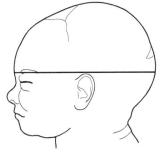

Figure 13.12 Upward moulding (dotted line) following persistent occipitoposterior position.

c. Figure 13.13 shows the head in a face presentation. Label the diameters, identify the length (cm) and colour in a dashed line to show the shape and direction of moulding.

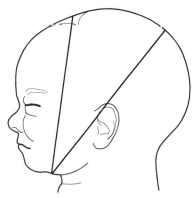

Figure 13.13 Moulding in a face presentation.

d. Figure 13.14 shows the head in a brow presentation. Label the diameter, identify the length (cm) and colour in a dashed line to show the direction of moulding.

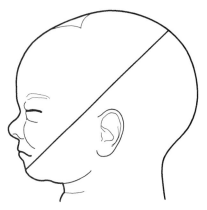

Figure 13.14 Moulding in a brow presentation.

Breech presentations

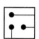 **Labelling**

14. Complete Figures 13.15–18 by labelling the four different types of breech presentations.

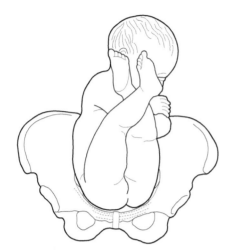

Figure 13.15

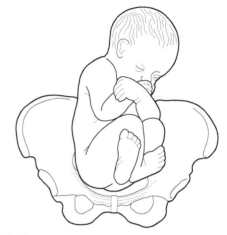

Figure 13.16

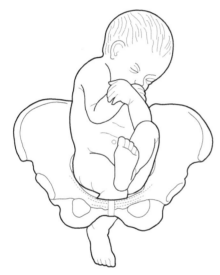

Figure 13.17

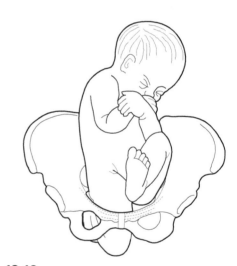

Figure 13.18

a. Figure 13.15 _____

b. Figure 13.16 _____

c. Figure 13.17 _____

d. Figure 13.18 _____

Completion

15. Complete Table 13.8 by inserting the correct missing word(s).

Table 13.8

	Mechanism of left sacroanterior position
a.	The lie is _____.
b.	The attitude is one of complete _____.
c.	The presentation is _____.
d.	The position is _____.
e.	The _____ is the sacrum.
f.	The presenting part is the _____.
g.	The _____ diameter (____ cm) enters the pelvis in the left oblique diameter of the brim. The _____ points to the iliopectineal eminence.

Breech births and manoeuvres

  Labelling and completion

16. Complete the following activities 16 (a–f) about breech births by using a combination of inserting a word(s) from the list provided and removing the incorrect word(s) to provide the correct information. Note that a few words may be used more than once.

ankles	flexion	neck	suboccipital
after-coming	fractured	occiput	symphysis pubis
arms	head	rotation	traction
chin	hypoxia	saggital	weight
crushed	legs	shoulders	vault
controlled	malar	stretch	

The following paragraphs relate to the birth of the head in a breech birth. Complete the paragraphs so that it reads correctly.

a. On birth of the _____ the baby is allowed to hang from the vulva **with/without**

support. The baby's _____ brings the head onto the pelvic floor on which the

_____ rotates. The _____ suture is now in the anteroposterior diameter

of the outlet. If the head does not **flex/rotate** then two fingers should be placed on the _____

bones and the head rotated. The baby can hang for up to 1 or 2 minutes. Gradually the _____

elongates, the hair-line appears and the _____ region can be felt. Three methods

used to achieve a controlled birth include: i. forceps applied to the _____

head; ii. Burns Marshall method and iii. Mauriceau-Smellie-Veit manoeuvre. Assistance is required for

babies born with extended _____ and extended _____.

_____ birth of the head is vital to avoid any sudden change in intracranial pressure.

b.   Complete the following Table 13.9.

Table 13.9

	Burns Marshall method (see Figure 13.19 for information)
i.	This method to control the birth of the head is conducted once the nape of the _____ and hairline are visible.
ii.	(A) in Figure 13.19. The baby is grasped by the **thighs/feet** and held **on stretch/relaxed**
iii.	(B) in Figure 13.19. The mouth and nose are free. The _____ of the head is delivered **slowly/quickly**.
iv.	The method involves the attendant standing facing **away from/towards** the mother. With the left hand, the attendant grasps the baby's _____ from behind with the forefinger between the two. The baby is kept on the _____ with sufficient **relaxation/traction** to prevent the neck from bending backwards and being _____. The _____ region, and not the neck, should pivot under the apex of the **perineum/pubic arch** or the spinal cord may be _____. The feet are taken up through an arc of 180° until the mouth and nose are free at the vulva.

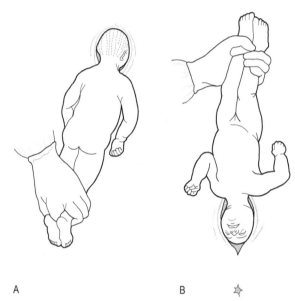

A   B   ✦

Figure 13.19 Burns Marshall method of delivering the after-coming head of a breech presentation: The baby is grasped by the feet and held on the stretch. The mouth and nose are free. The vault of the head is delivered slowly.

c. Complete Table 13.10.

Table 13.10

	Mauriceau-Smellie-Veit manoeuvre (see Figure 13.20 for information)
i.	Mauriceau-Smellie-Veit manoeuvre is mainly used when there is delay in descent of the head because of **flexion/extension**. The manoeuvre promotes jaw **extension/flexion** and shoulder **extension/traction**.
ii.	(A) in Figure 13.20. The hands are in position **after/before** the body is lifted.
iii.	(B) in Figure 13.20. This shows extraction of the _____.
iv.	The manoeuvre involves the baby being laid astride the **fingers/arm** with the palm supporting the **head/chest**. One finger is placed on each _____ bone to flex the _____. The middle finger may be used to apply pressure to the _____. Two fingers of the attendant's other hand are hooked over the shoulders with the middle finger pushing up the _____ to aid _____. _____ is applied to draw the head out of the vagina and, when the _____ region appears, the body is lifted to assist the head to pivot around the _____. The _____ is delivered **quickly/slowly**.

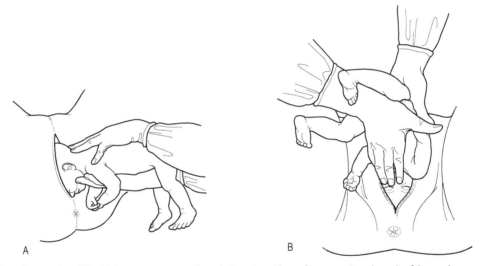

A   B

Figure 13.20 Mauriceau–Smellie–Veit manoeuvre for delivering the after-coming head of breech presentation: The hands are in position before the body is lifted. Extraction of the head.

d. Complete Table 13.11.

Table 13.11

Extended Legs (see Figure 13.21 for information)
When the popliteal fossae appear at the vulva, **four/two** fingers are placed along the length of one thigh with the fingertips **on the ankle/in the fossa**. The leg is swept to the side of the abdomen (**adducting/abducting** the **hip/knee**) and the knee is **deflexed/flexed** by the pressure on its under surface and the **upper/lower** part of the leg will emerge from the vagina. The process is repeated for the other leg.

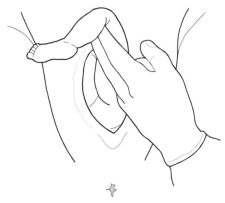

Figure 13.21

e. Complete the following activities related to the Loveset manoeuvre for delivery of extended arms. Figure 13.22 shows the correct grasp and Figure 13.23 details the manoeuvre.

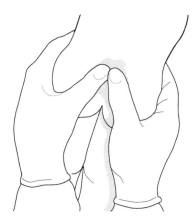

Figure 13.22

In Figure 13.23 insert an arrow in each diagram to correctly position the direction of rotation and/or downward traction in this manoeuvre.

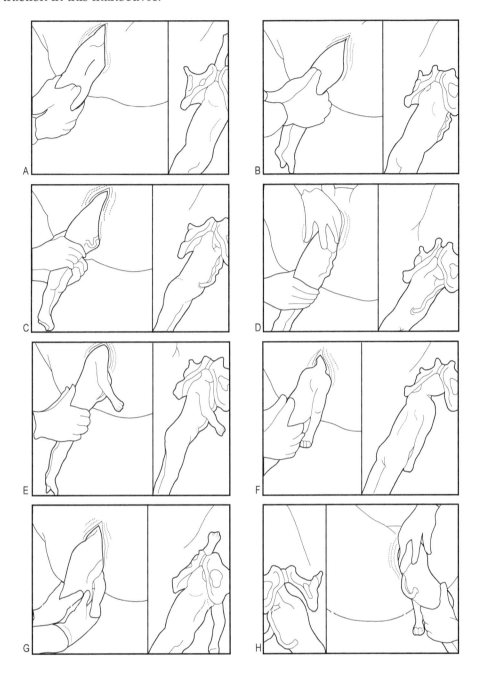

Figure 13.23 This figure details Loveset manoeuvre. In each diagram above (A–H) insert a bold arrow to show the direction of rotation and/or downward traction in this manoeuvre.

f. Complete Table 13.12.

Table 13.12

	Loveset manoeuvre (see Figure 13.23 for information)
i.	This manoeuvre involves a combination of _____ and **upward/downward** traction to deliver the **legs/arms**. The direction of _____ must always bring the **back/abdomen** uppermost and the arms are delivered from under the pubic arch. This manoeuvre needs to be conducted promptly to avoid any further delay and possible _____.

? Pot luck multiple choice questions (MCQs)

17. Occipitoposterior position occurs in approximately:

   a. 5% of labours

   b. 10% of labours

   c. 15% of labours

   d. 20% of labours

18. A persistent occipitoposterior position results from failure of internal rotation prior to birth. The incidence of births is:

   a. 1%   b. 5%   c. 10%   d. 15%

19. The incidence of shoulder presentation near term is approximately:

   a. 1: 100 pregnancies

   b. 1: 300 pregnancies

   c. 1: 500 pregnancies

   d. 1: 700 pregnancies

20. The most common cause of shoulder presentation is due to:

   a. Contracted pelvis

   b. Low uterine fibroid

   c. Lax abdominal and uterine muscles

   d. Cervical fibroid

21. If on abdominal examinations the lie tends to vary then it is defined as unstable lie after:

   a. 32 weeks' gestation

   b. 34 weeks' gestation

   c. 36 weeks' gestation

   d. 38 weeks' gestation

Reference

NICE (2008) Intrapartum Care Guideline. [Online] Available at: http://www.nice.org.uk/guidance/CG70/NICEGuidance [Accessed 24 April 2012].

CHAPTER 14 Midwifery and obstetric emergencies

This chapter focuses on midwifery and obstetric emergencies. Assisted births will also be included. Recognizing signs and symptoms of the problem and immediate action is vital and may determine the outcome for the mother and fetus. The activities will test your knowledge in a variety of emergency situations.

True/false

1. Consider the following statements in Table 14.1. Complete the table by deciding if the statements are correct by ticking the appropriate column.

Table 14.1

	Statement	True	False
a.	Bradycardia, and variable or prolonged decelerations of the fetal heart are associated with cord compression.		
b.	Shoulder dystocia is a soft tissue dystocia.		
c.	Occult cord prolapse occurs when the cord lies in front of the presenting part.		
d.	The foot of the bed is raised in the Trendelenburg position.		
e.	In shoulder dystocia, traction will promote attempts at delivery.		
f.	Gaskin manoeuvre is another term for the 'all-four position'.		
g.	Once cord prolapsed is diagnosed then an oxytocin infusion in progress should be stopped.		
h.	Shoulder dystocia is not a common emergency.		

Cord prolapse

Short answers

2. This activity relates to the positions adopted in the emergency situation of 'cord prolapse'. Figures 14.1 and 14.2 show two different positions. Complete the following related questions.

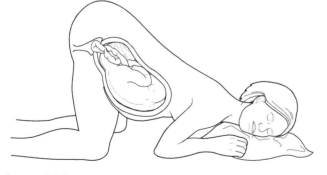

Figure 14.2

Figure 14.1

    a. Name the position adopted in Figure 14.1: _____

    b. Name the position adopted in Figure 14.2: _____

c. What is the key purpose for adopting these positions? _____

_____

d. What other action can the midwife take to achieve the same purpose? _____

_____

✏️ Completion

3. This activity relates to the immediate action of the midwife on diagnosis of the emergency situation of cord prolapse. Complete the statements by inserting the missing word(s) and numerical value.

a. Call for assistance and note the _____.

b. If the cord lies outside the vagina, then it should be gently _____ to prevent

_____, to maintain _____ and prevent _____.

c. Oxygen may be administered to the mother by face mask at _____ L/min and this may improve fetal

_____.

d. The midwife may need to keep her _____ in the _____ and hold the

_____ off the umbilical cord, especially during a _____

_____.

e. Birth must be expedited with the greatest possible speed. Three modes of birth are possible depending on

circumstances: i. Birth will be by _____ if the fetus is alive but vaginal birth

is not imminent. ii. Birth may be by _____ with the midwife performing an

_____ if the cord prolapse is diagnosed in second stage (multiparous mother).

iii. Where the presentation is cephalic, birth may be assisted and achieved through _____

or _____.

Shoulder dystocia

↰ ✎ Matching and completion

4. Complete the following paragraph by inserting words chosen from the list provided so that it reads correctly.

anterior	hollow	pelvis	sacral promontory
behind	impactation	posterior	symphysis pubis
gravity	inlet	sacrum	uterus

Shoulder dystocia occurs when the _____ shoulder becomes trapped _____ or

on the _____, while the _____ shoulder may be in the

_____ of the _____ or high above the _____.

In shoulder dystocia, the _____ is at the pelvic _____ and the force of

_____ will keep the fetus against the mother's _____ and _____.

✎ Completion

5. **HELPERR** mnemonic is used as a prompt for midwives to aid them with the systematic series of actions and manoeuvres applied to disimpact the shoulders. Complete the following mnemonic by inserting the appropriate actions taken by the midwife at each stage.

   H: _____ for _____.

   E: _____ need assessed.

   L: _____ position.

   P: _____.

   E: _____ (internal rotation).

   R: _____ _____ arm

   R: _____ and try again.

6. Complete the following terminology by removing the incorrect word.

   a. The term 'adduct' means to pull or move something (e.g. arm or leg) **towards/away from** the midline of the body or a toe or finger **towards/away from** the axis of the leg or arm.

   b. The term 'abduct' means to pull or move something (e.g. arm or leg) **towards/away from** the midline of the body or a toe or finger **towards/away from** the axis of the leg or arm.

Positions and manoeuvres used in shoulder dystocia

  Matching and completion

7. Figures 14.3 and 14.4 show positions and manoeuvres that may be involved in shoulder dystocia. Table 14.2 provides an activity related to non-invasive procedures. Complete the table by: i. answering the question, ii. inserting the missing word(s) from the list provided and iii. removing the incorrect word(s).

hollow   pressure   sacral promontory   symphysis pubis

posterior   sacrum   suprapubic pressure   weight

Table 14.2

	Non-invasive procedures
a.	Name the position shown in Figure 14.3 _____ This manoeuvre will **diminish/rotate** the angle of the _____ superiorly and use the _____ of the mother's legs to create gentle _____ on her abdomen, releasing the impaction of the **anterior/posterior** shoulder.
b.	What action does Figure 14.4 demonstrate? _____ Pressure should be exerted on the side of the fetal **chest/back** and towards the fetal **chest/back**. This manoeuvre may help to **adduct/abduct** the shoulders and push the **anterior/posterior** shoulder away from the _____ into the larger oblique or transverse diameter.
c.	The 'all fours position' may be especially helpful if the _____ shoulder is impacted behind the _____ as this position optimizes space available in the sacral curve and may allow the _____ shoulder to be delivered first.

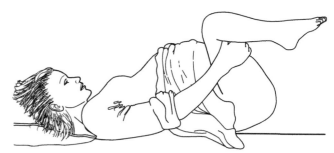

Figure 14.3

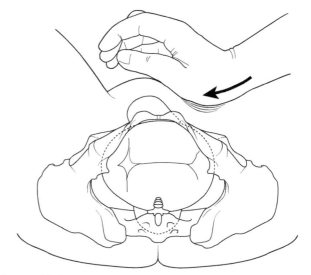

Figure 14.4

8. Figures 14.5–14.7 show positions and manoeuvres that may be involved in shoulder dystocia. Table 14.3 provides an activity related to manipulative procedures. Complete the table by inserting the missing word(s) from the list provided in question 7 or by removing the incorrect word(s).

Table 14.3

	Manipulative procedures
a.	Name the manoeuvre shown in Figure 14.5 _____ In this manoeuvre, the midwife on VE needs to identify the **anterior/posterior** shoulder. Then the **anterior/posterior** shoulder is pushed in the direction of the fetal **chest/back**, thus rotating the **anterior/posterior** shoulder away from the _____. **Adducting/abducting** the shoulders reduces the 12 cm bisacromial diameter.
b.	Name the manoeuvre shown in Figure 14.6 _____ In this manoeuvre, the midwife inserts her hand into the vagina and identifies the fetal **chest/back**. Pressure is exerted on the **posterior/anterior** fetal shoulder achieving rotation. This manoeuvre **abducts/adducts** the shoulders and also rotates the shoulders into a more favourable diameter for birth.

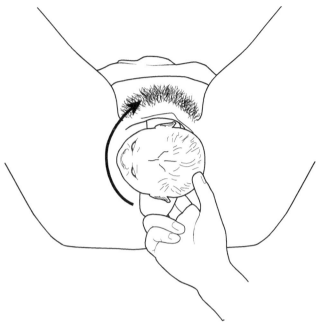

Figure 14.5

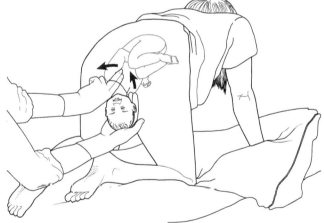

Figure 14.6

Continued →

Table 14.3 contiued

	Manipulative procedures
c.	Figure 14.7 (A–D) shows delivery of the posterior arm. This manoeuvre makes use of the space created by the _____ of the _____ (as seen in A and B). Figure C shows two fingers splinting the **humerus/shoulder** of the **anterior/posterior** arm. Figure D shows the elbow **flexed/extended** and the forearm being swept over the **chest/back** to deliver the hand.

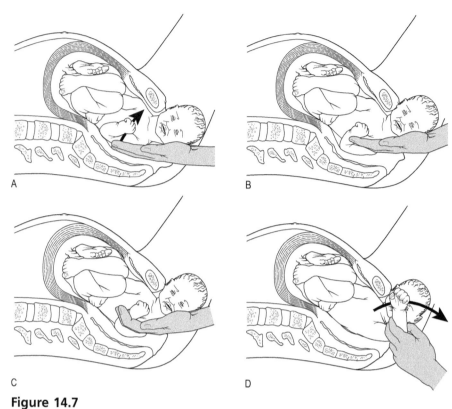

A　　　　　　　　　　　B

C　　　　　　　　　　　D

Figure 14.7

Rupture of the uterus and inversion of the uterus

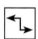 **Matching and completion**

9. Rupture of the uterus is one of the most serious complications in midwifery and obstetrics. Complete the following Table 14.4 by matching the statements correctly to the most likely type of uterine rupture (i–iii).

  i. Complete rupture of the uterus   ii. Incomplete rupture of the uterus   iii. Dehiscence (bursting) of an existing scar

Table 14.4

	Statements
a.	This rupture involves tearing of the uterine wall but not the perimetrium.
b.	Rupture occurring along the fibrous scar tissue (avascular) may result in scantly blood loss.　　　　and
c.	This involves rupture of the uterine wall but the fetal membranes remain intact.
d.	This type of rupture in a non-scarred uterus may present with sudden collapse of the mother who complains of severe abdominal pain.
e.	This rupture involves a tear in the wall of the uterus with or without expulsion of the fetus.

10. Consider the statements related to inversion of the uterus in Table 14.5. Complete the table by matching the statements to the classification of inversion of the uterus (i–vi).

i. First-degree   ii. Second-degree   iii. Third-degree
iv. Acute   v. Subacute   vi. Chronic

Table 14.5

	Statement
a.	This occurs within the first 24 hours.
b.	The body or the corpus of the uterus is inverted to the internal os.
c.	This occurs after the first 24 hours and within 4 weeks.
d.	The fundus reaches the internal os.
e.	This occurs after 4 weeks
f.	The uterus, cervix and vagina are inverted and visible.

Instrumental and operative births

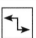 **Matching and completion**

11. Consider the statements related to types of forceps/ventouse in Table 14.6. Complete the table by matching the statements to obstetric forceps/ventouse (i–iv).

i. Wrigley's forceps   ii. Keilland's forceps
iii. Neville-Barnes or Simpson's forceps   iv. Ventouse

Table 14.6

	Statements
a.	These are generally used for a low or mid cavity delivery when the sagittal suture is in the anteroposterior diameter of the cavity/outlet of the pelvis. _____.
b.	These are generally used for rotation and extraction of the head that is arrested in the deep transverse or in the occipitoposterior position. _____.
c.	This is associated with more incidences of cephalohaematoma than other facial and cranial injuries. _____.
d.	These are also used for the after-coming head of a breech delivery, or at a caesarean section. _____.
e.	This involves positioning over the sagittal suture. _____.
f.	These are designed to be used when the head is on the perineum. _____.
g.	This cleaves to the baby's scalp by suction. _____.

12. The following activity relates to the sequence of anatomical layers involved in the operative procedure of caesarean section. Complete the activity using the list provided by inserting the correct sequence commencing with the outer layer of skin.

Abdominal peritoneum   Muscle (rectus abdominis)   Rectus sheath

Fat   Pelvic peritoneum   Uterine muscle

Skin → _____ → _____

→ _____ → _____

→ _____ → _____

Shock – classification and physiology

 Matching

13. Consider the statements related to 'shock' in Table 14.7. Complete the table by matching the statements to the classification of shock (i–v).

    i. Hypovolaemic   ii. Cardiogeneic   iii. Neurogenic

    iv. Septic or toxic   v. Anaphylactic

Table 14.7

	Statement
a.	This may occur as a result of severe allergy or drug reaction. _____.
b.	This results from an insult to the nervous system. _____.
c.	This results from a reduction in intravascular volume. _____.
d.	This is due to impaired ability of the heart to pump blood. _____.
e.	This occurs with a severe generalized infection. _____.

 Completion

14. The following activity relates to 'shock'. Complete the following paragraph by inserting the correct missing word from the list provided.

acute	complex	inadequate	organ
chronic	death	multisystem	tissues
circulatory	failure	recovery	
collapse	fatal	reduction	

Shock is a _____ syndrome involving a _____ in blood flow to the _____ that may

result in irreversible _____ damage and progressive _____ of the _____

system. If left untreated it will result in _____.

Shock can be _____ but prompt treatment results in _____ with little detrimental effect on the

mother. However _____ treatment or _____ to initiate effective treatment can result in a

_____ condition ending in _____ organ failure which may be _____.

 Completion

15. Table 14.8 lists the types of 'shock'. Complete the table by inserting one example of the possible cause of each type of shock. If relevant, provide an one example related to obstetrics.

Table 14.8

	Type	Possible cause
a.	Hypovolaemic	
b.	Anaphylactic	
c.	Neurogenic	
d.	Septic or toxic	
e.	Cardiogenic	

16. The following two activities relate to the physiological effects of 'shock'. Complete the activities by removing the incorrect word(s) so that the paragraph reads correctly:

a. This paragraph relates to the compensatory stage of hypovolaemic shock.

The **rise/drop** in cardiac output produces a response from the **sympathetic/peripheral** nervous system through the activation of receptors in the **aorta and carotid arteries/renal arteries**. Blood is redistributed to the **vital organs/skin**. There is **constriction/dilatation** of the vessel in the gastrointestinal tract, kidneys, skin, and lungs. Peristalsis **slows/increases**, urinary output is **increased/reduced** and exchange of gas is impaired as blood flow **increases/diminishes**. The heart rate **decreases/increases** and the pupils of the eyes **constrict/dilate**. Sweat glands are **stimulated/inactive** and the skin becomes **dry and warm/moist and clammy**. Adrenaline (Epinephrine) is released from the adrenal **medulla/cortex** and aldosterone from the adrenal **medulla/cortex**. Antidiuretic hormone (ADH) is secreted from the **anterior/posterior** lobe of the pituitary gland. Their combined effect is to cause **vasoconstriction/vasodilatation**, **decreased/increased** cardiac output and a **decrease/increase** in urinary output. Venous return to the heart will **increase/decrease** but this will not be sustained unless the fluid loss is replaced.

b. This paragraph relates to 'adult respiratory distress syndrome' (ARDS) due to the physiological effects 'shock' has on the lungs.

Gas exchange is **impaired/unaffected** as the physiological dead space **increases/decreases** within the lungs. Levels of carbon dioxide **rise/fall** and arterial oxygen levels **fall/remain unchanged**. **Ischaemia/increased blood flow** within the lungs alters the production of **surfactant/renin** and as a result of this, alveoli **collapse/enlarge**. Oedema in the lungs, due to **increased/decreased** permeability, **exacerbates/reduces** the existing problem of diffusion of oxygen. Atelectasis, oedema and **reduced/increased** compliance impair ventilation and gaseous exchange. This leads ultimately to respiratory **failure/improvement**.

Amniotic fluid embolism

 Completion

17. Complete the following paragraph related to amniotic fluid embolism by inserting the missing word and by removing the incorrect word(s) so that it reads correctly.

Amniotic fluid embolism occurs when amniotic fluid enters the **maternal** circulation via the

_____ or _____ site. Maternal collapse can be **rapidly/insidiously**

progressive. The body's initial response is pulmonary **vasospasm/vasodilation** causing hypoxia, **hypertension/**

hypotension, _____ oedema and cardiovascular collapse. Secondly there is the development of

left/right ventricular failure, with haemorrhage and _____ disorder and further uncontrollable

_____. There is uterine **hypertonus/hypotonus** and this will induce fetal

_____ in response to uterine _____.

18. Table 14.9 relates to maternal signs and symptoms of amniotic fluid embolism. Complete the missing information by answering the questions and inserting the missing signs and symptoms.

Table 14.9

	Maternal signs and symptoms of amniotic fluid embolism
a.	Cardiovascular? Pulse rate: _____ Blood pressure: _____ Peripheral circulation effects: _____ • Severe effects: Cardiac arrest.
b.	Respiratory? Colour: _____ Breathing: _____ • Severe effects: Respiratory arrest.
c.	Haematological? • Coagulation disorders/DIC. What happens at the placental site? _____, where required. _____
d.	Neurological? What is the mother acting like? _____ What may the mother experience? _____ • Pain is less likely.

Basic life support measures

19. Complete the following activities by providing the missing information to complete the statements in Table 14.10 relating to basic life support measures. Always refer to updated resuscitation guidelines.

Table 14.10

	Statement
a.	Shake and _____
b.	Call for _____
c.	A – _____ Check for chest _____
d.	B – _____ Listen for _____
e.	C – _____ Check for _____
f.	Appropriate position for body: _____ Precaution for pregnancy: _____
g.	Position for head: _____
h.	Use _____ compressions : _____ breaths
i.	Continue until _____

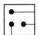 **Colour and labelling**

20. Figure 14.8 shows cricoids pressure and the related structures. Complete the activity by colouring and labelling as noted.

Colour and label

Adam's apple
Oesophagus
Cricoids cartilage
Trachea

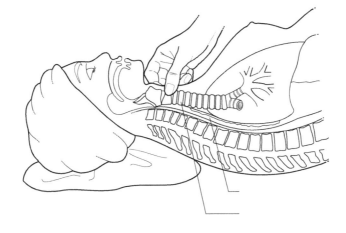

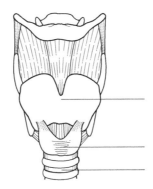

Figure 14.8

 Multiple choice questions (MCQs)

21. In a cord prolapse, the bladder can be filled with 500–700 mL of sterile saline which elevates the presenting part above the ischial spines by about:

    a. 0.5 cm   b. 1 cm   c. 2 cm   d. 4 cm

22. The incidence of acute inversion of the uterus is approximately:

    a. 1 in 5000 births

    b. 1 in 10 000 births

    c. 1 in 15 000 births

    d. 1 in 20 000 births

23. Central venous pressure (CVP) is the pressure in the:

    a. Pulmonary artery

    b. Left atrium or inferior vena cava

    c. Pulmonary vein

    d. Right atrium or superior vena cava

24. The normal central pressure varies between:

    a.   20 and 25 cm of H_2O

    b.   15 and 20 cm of H_2O

    c.   10 and 15 cm of H_2O

    d.   5 and 10 cm of H_2O

25. In shock the CVP pressure will be persistently:

    a.   Low and below 5 cm of H_2O

    b.   Low and below 10 cm of H_2O

    c.   High and above 15 cm of H_2O

    d.   High and above 25 cm of H_2O

CHAPTER 15 The puerperium

This chapter focuses on the physiology of the puerperium and also includes physical and psychological complications. The anatomy of the breasts and the physiology of lactation are included. The activities will test your knowledge in these areas.

Short answers and completion

1. Complete the following definitions/statements by inserting the missing word(s).

   a. The puerperium starts immediately after delivery of the _____ and _____ and

   continues for _____ weeks (in the absence of complications). It is expected that by this time all the

   _____ _____ will have recovered from the effects of pregnancy and returned to their ____–

   _____ state.

   (N.B. It is now professionally recognized that some women continue to experience problems related to childbirth that extend well beyond the defined period of puerperium above and the possibility of a longer duration is now accepted alongside the range of initial morbidity).

   b. The postnatal period is defined in the UK as _____

   _____

   _____ (NMC 2004).

   c. Following birth, there are changes in the levels of circulating pregnancy related hormones that

   impact on the puerperium. Recap on these hormones which include: i. _____,

   ii. _____, iii. _____,

   iv. _____.

Uterine Changes

 Completion

2. This activity relates to the physiological processes taking place in the uterus at the end of third stage. Complete the activity by inserting the missing word(s) from the extended list provided. A few words may be used more than once. You should insert the numerical values required.

anterior	epithelium	phagocytic	thrombin
autolysis	firm	posterior	thromboplastin
below	ischaemia	prolactin	vasoconstriction
blood loss	ischaemic	proteolytic	posterior
centrally	ligatures	reduction	thrombin
coagulation	macrophages	renal	
contraction	myometrium	sinuses	

On expulsion of the placenta and membranes, the muscle layers of the _____ simulate the action

of _____ that compress and occlude the large _____ of the blood vessels exposed by

placental separation to reduce _____. In addition, de-oxygenation and a state of

_____ arise in tissues due to _____ in the overall blood supply to the

uterus. Through the process of _____, autodigestion of the _____ muscle fibres by

_____ enzymes occurs resulting in an overall _____ in their size. There is

_____ action of polymorphs and _____ in the blood and lymphatic systems

upon the waste products of autolysis, which are then excreted via the _____ system in the urine.

_____ takes place through platelet aggregation and the release of _____

and fibrin.

   Apart from the placental site, what remains of the inner surface of the uterine lining, regenerates rapidly to

produce a covering of _____. Partial covering occurs within ___–____ days after birth; total

coverage is complete by the ____st day.

   Once the placenta has separated, there is a _____ in the circulating levels of hormones related

to pregnancy. This leads to further physiological changes in muscle and connective tissue as well as having a

major influence on the secretion of _____ from the _____ pituitary gland.

On initial abdominal palpation the fundus of the uterus should be located _____, its position being

at the same level or slightly _____ the umbilicus and should feel _____ to confirm it is in a state of

_____.

Infection in the puerperium

 Completion

3. In the event that a woman following birth is unwell, is pale and listless, has a temperature and has a tachycardia then this would indicate that she may have an infection. Complete the following activity in Table 15.1 by inserting the missing word(s) related to the possible findings the midwife may note on postnatal examination.

Table 15.1

	Site	Possible findings
a.	Uterus	On palpation the uterus may be _____ contracted and feel wide and '_____'. This might be described as '_____ - involution'. The fundus may be _____ to one side and not progressively _____ in size. The woman may experience _____ on palpation. When compared with the findings from a previous examination, _____ loss may be fresher and _____ or _____ but _____ smelling. The woman may pass _____.
b.	Wounds	There may be: _____ and tenderness around a wound area. _____ healing or _____ at the skin edges. _____ felt deeper in the wound area (as experienced by the woman). Virulent clear or _____ exudate.
c.	Breasts	May feel tight and _____. One segment may be flushed or _____. One or both nipples may have _____, broken or /discoloured/flaky skin.

True/false

4. Consider the following statements in Table 15.2. Complete the table by deciding if the statements are correct by ticking the appropriate column.

Table 15.2

	Statement	True	False
a.	Afterpains and uterine tenderness on palpation should not be defined as separate issues.		
b.	Just after birth, the major constitutes of vaginal loss is blood products.		
c.	Retained placental fragments and other products of conception are likely to inhibit the process of involution.		
d.	The most common species associated with puerperal sepsis is the ß-haemolytic S. pyogenes (Lancefield group A).		
e.	As involution progresses, vaginal loss contains stale blood, lanugo, vernix and other unwanted products of conception.		
f.	Hormonal influences seem to be implicated in the postnatal 'blues'.		
g.	Psychiatric disorders are associated with a decrease in fertility.		

The breasts and breastfeeding

  Colouring and labelling

5. Figure 15.1 shows the cross section of the breast. Colour and label the figure as noted.

Colour and label

Glandular tissue
Main milk ducts converging to enter the nipple
Areola margin
Fat is behind the breast interspersed between glandular tissue, and just under the skin
Milk duct

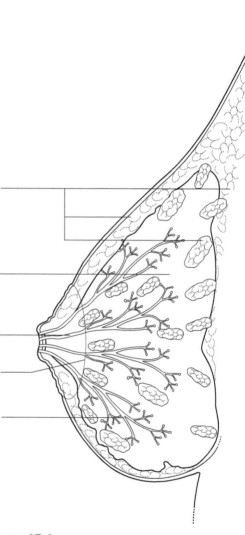

Figure 15.1

 Completion

6. Complete the following activity relating to the physiology of breastfeeding by inserting the missing word(s) from the list provided.

acini	fuller	lobe	oxytocin
accumulates	inhibit	milk removal	prolactin
autocrine inhibitory factor	lactiferous ducts	myoepithelial	shorter
distends	lactiferous tubules	negative feedback control	stepped up
ductal	longitudinally	nipple	whey protein

The alveoli contain _____ cells, which produce milk and are surrounded by _____ cells which contract and propel the milk out. Small _____, carrying milk from the alveoli, unite to form larger ducts. Several large ducts (_____) conveying milk from one or more _____ emerge on the surface of the _____. _____ cells are orientated _____ along the ducts and, under the influence of _____, these smooth muscle cells contract and the tubule becomes _____ and wider. The tubule _____ during active milk flow, while the _____ cells are maintained in a state of contracting by circulating _____ (2–3 min). The _____ the breast when let down occurs, the greater the degree of _____ distension.

As lactation progresses, the _____ response to suckling diminishes and _____ _____ becomes the driving force behind milk production. This is due to _____ in secreted milk that is able to _____ the synthesis of milk constituents. This protein accumulates in the breast as the milk _____ and it exerts _____ on the continued production of milk. Removal of this _____ by removing the milk, allows milk production to be _____ again. This is sometimes referred to as feedback inhibitor of lactation (FIL).

True/false

7. Table 15.3 provides statements related to breast and breastfeeding. Complete the activity by deciding if the statements are true or false by ticking the appropriate column.

Table 15.3

	Statement	True	False
a.	The nipple is covered with epithelium and contains smooth muscle and elastic fibres.		
b.	Prolactin seems to be much more important to the continuation of lactation than to its initiation.		
c.	Milk release is under neuroendocrine control.		
d.	Montgomery's glands produce a sebum-like substance which acts as a lubricant during pregnancy and breastfeeding.		
e.	In the early days of lactation, the 'let down' or 'milk ejection' reflex is conditioned.		
f.	Prolactin is not involved in the suppression of ovulation.		
g.	Healthy breastfeeding women undertaking strenuous exercise (from 6–8 weeks after birth) will not affect either the quality or quantity of milk.		
h.	Milk production is affected by fluctuations in the mother's fluid intake.		
i.	Tactile stimulation of the breast stimulates oxytocin release.		
j.	Expressed human milk can be stored for up to 2 weeks in the freezer compartment of a fridge.		

Breastmilk

 Completion

8. The following activity relates to the constituents of human milk. Complete the following statements by inserting the correct word(s) from the list provided. A few words may be used more than once.

bifidus factor	foremilk	lactoferrin
blood-clotting	higher	lactose
calcium	highest	lowest
colostrum	hindmilk	low fat
curds	IgA	mucosal
decreases	immunoglobulins	protein
E. coli	increase	rapidly
fat	lactobacilli	whey
fat soluble	*Lactobacillus bifidus*	

a. Colostrum has a _____ fat and protein content than mature milk.

b. _____ (at the beginning of the feed) is of a high volume of relatively _____

milk. _____ (as the feed progresses) _____ in volume with an

_____ in the proportion of fat sometimes by as much as five times the initial value.

c. It is the _____ content and not the _____ that has particular significance for the

_____ growing brain of the newborn. The fat content is _____ in the morning and

_____ in the afternoon.

d. The main carbohydrate component is provided by _____ (which provides the baby with

about 40% calorific requirements). This enhances the absorption of _____ and promotes the

growth of _____ which _____ intestinal acidity thus reducing the growth of

pathogenic organisms.

e. The dominant protein is _____ which forms soft, flocculent _____ when acidified in the

stomach.

f. The _____ promotes the growth of Gram-positive bacilli in the gut flora,

particularly _____, which discourages the multiplication of pathogens.

_____ binds to enteric iron, preventing pathogenic _____ from obtaining the

iron needed for them to survive.

g. All the vitamins required for good nutrition and health are supplied in breastmilk.

_____ vitamin K is present in milk and is essential for the synthesis of

_____ factors. It is present in greater concentrations in _____ and

in the high fat _____.

h. _____ are present to provide protection. The most important for the baby is

_____ which covers the intestinal epithelium and protects the _____ surfaces against

pathogenic bacteria and enteroviruses.

Breastfeeding complications

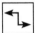 **Matching**

9. Consider the statements related to breast problems in Table 15.4. Complete the table by matching the statements to the most likely breast problem.

i. Breast abcess	ii. Blocked ducts	iii. *Candida albicans* (thrush)
iv. Engorgement	v. Epithelial overgrowth	vi. Mastitis
vii. Sore and damaged nipples	viii. White spots	

Table 15.4

	Statements
a.	Breasts are hard, often oedematous, painful and sometimes flushed. It occurs around day 3 or 4.
b.	A fluctuant swelling may develop in a previously inflamed area. Pus may be discharged from the nipple.
c.	A ductal opening in the tip of the nipple is obstructed by a white granule or by epithelial growth. This is not common.
d.	The mother feels lumpy areas in the breast due to distended glandular tissue. Breasts may be firm, tender and possibly flushed.
e.	This is a more common cause of a physical obstruction. A white blister is evident on the surface of the nipple closing off one of the exit points in the nipple.
f.	This is often the result of milk stasis. There is inflammation in the breast with typically one or more adjacent segments inflamed and appears as a wedge-shaped area of redness or swelling. It is mainly non-infective but can also be infective.
g.	The cause is almost always due to trauma from the baby's mouth and tongue.
h.	This is not common in the first week. The nipple and areola appear inflamed and shiny. Sudden onset of pain in a trouble-free period of feeding. Pain persists through the feed.

? Multiple choice questions (MCQs)

10. Colostrum is present in pregnancy from:

    a. 6th week   b. 10th week   c. 16th week   d. 20th week

11. If breastfeeding (or expressing) is delayed, lactation can still be initiated (due to high prolactin levels) for at least:

    a. 2 days   b. 4 days   c. 7 days   d. 14 days

12. Calcium is more efficiently absorbed from human milk because of the:

    a. Lower calcium: phosphorus ratio

    b. Higher phosphorus content

    c. Higher calcium: phosphorus ratio

    d. None of the above

13. NICE (2008) advises that expressed breastmilk can be stored in the main part of a fridge, at 4°C or lower for:

    a. Up to 2 days

    b. Up to 5 days

    c. Up to 8 days

    d. Up to 10 days

14. Which of the following infective organisms are endogenous (already present in/on the body):

    a. *Chlamydia trachomatis*

    b. *Escherichia coli*

    c. *Clostridium welchii*

    d. a and b

    e. b and c

15. The prevalence of psychiatric disorder (current or previous) in young women in early pregnancy is:

    a. 5%   b. 10%   c. 15%   d. 20%

16. The incidence of postnatal women developing a depressive illness is approximately:

    a. 5%   b. 10%   c. 15%   d. 20%

17. The recurrence of puerperal psychosis (the most severe form of postpartum affective disorder) in future pregnancies is:

    a. 10%   b. 20%   c. 30%   d. 50%

18. Which method of contraception is not recommended for lactating mothers:

    a. Progestogen oral pill

    b. Progestogen implants

    c. Combined oral contraception

    d. Progestogen-releasing intrauterine system (IUS)

References

NICE (2008) PH 11 Maternal and Child Nutrition: Guidance. [Online] Available at: http://guidance.nice.org.uk/PH11/Guidance/pdf/English [Accessed 24 April 2012].

NMC (2004) Midwives rules and standards. [Online] Available at: http://www.nmc-uk.org/Publications/Standards/ [Accessed 24 April 2012].

CHAPTER

16 Complementary therapies and pharmacology in childbirth

This chapter focuses on complementary therapies and pharmacology in childbirth. The midwife needs to have knowledge of current practice and how these impact on the woman and fetus. The activities will test your knowledge in these areas.

COMPLEMENTARY THERAPIES

Classifications of complementary therapies

 Matching

1. Table 16.1 presents the three classifications of complementary or alternative therapies used in the UK. Complete the table by matching the list of therapies appropriately within the correct classification group.

1. Acupuncture	2. Alexander technique	3. Anthroposophical medicine	4. Aromatherapy
5. Bach flower remedies	6. Chiropractic	7. Crystal therapies	8. Dowsing
9. Herbal medicine	10. Homeopathy	11. Hypnotherapy/ hypnosis	12. Indian Ayurvedic medicine
13. Iridology	14. Japanese kampo	15. Kinesiology	16. Massage
17. Naturopathy	18. Nutritional therapies	19. Oesteopathy	20. Radionics
21. Reflexology/reflex zone therapy	22. Reiki	23. Shiatsu	24. Stress management
25. Traditional Chinese medicine (TCM)	26. Tibetan medicine	27. Yoga	

Table 16.1

	Groups of therapies
a.	**Group 1** therapies are professionally organized, complete systems of healthcare with national standards of education, statutory or voluntary self-regulation, disciplinary codes of practice and a reasonable body of evidence. These include the following therapies: _____ _____
b.	**Group 2** therapies are complementary or supportive to other healthcare, with less available evidence, many therapies are in the process of regulatory development and most organizations have chosen voluntary self-regulation. These include the following therapies: _____ _____ _____
c.	**Group 3** therapies are alternative, largely unregulated therapies with little or no body of evidence and divided into two sub-groups: a. traditional systems; b. diagnostic therapies. These include the following therapies: **Group 3a** – traditional systems: _____ _____ **Group 3b** – diagnostic therapies: _____ _____

Complementary therapies in pregnancy and childbirth

True/false

2. Consider the following statements in Table 16.2 relating to complementary therapies in pregnancy and childbirth. Complete the table by deciding if the statements are correct by ticking the appropriate column.

Table 16.2

	Statement	True	False
a.	Culinary use of herbs and herbal teas are generally safe in normal amounts.		
b.	Essential oils can be administered via the skin, respiratory tract, mucus membranes and the gastrointestinal tract.		
c.	Pregnant women often have very rapid and very profound reactions to reflexology.		
d.	Ginger biscuits should be advised as a remedy for nausea.		
e.	Raspberry leaf tea is thought to facilitate normal uterine action.		
f.	Essential oils and pharmaceutical drugs are absorbed, metabolized and excreted via separate biochemical pathways.		
g.	The use of essential oils is contraindicated with neonates as it may interfere with the mother/infant bonding process.		
h.	When inhaled, essential oil molecules reach the limbic centre in the brain, the circulation and major organs.		
i.	Homeopathic remedies interfere with breastfeeding.		

Completion

3. The use of moxibustion for breech presentation is gaining popularity in the UK. Complete the following related paragraph by removing the incorrect word(s) so that it reads correctly.

The herb used in this technique is a stick of dried **mugwort/yarrow**. This is used as a **heat/cold** source over **Bladder/Spleen** 67 acupuncture point on the **inner/outer** edges of the **little/big** toes. This is thought to stimulate **thyroid/adrenocortical** output which causes a **decrease/increase** in placental lactogens and changes in **oestrogens/prostaglandins**. Myometrial sensitivity and contractility is **decreased/increased**. In turn the fetal heart rate **increases/decreases** and there is an **increase/decrease** in fetal **breathing/movements.** This causes the fetus to turn so that the breech is in the **upper/lower** pole of the uterus and the cephalic is in the **upper/lower** pole of the uterus. The procedure is normally done around **34–35 weeks'/36–37 weeks'** gestation and performed on **one foot/ two feet** for **15/45** min, twice daily for up to **5 days/10 days**.

4. Cabbage leaves are well known as a method of easing breast engorgement. Complete the following paragraph on the related advice by inserting the correct words from the list provided.

chemical	damp	new	washed
chlorophyll	dark green	osmosis	white
comfort	drawing off	relief	wiped clean

From the literature, it is generally thought that the most effective leaves for easing engorgement are the

_____ cabbage leaves (only one study has found the _____ cabbage leaves more

effective). This is caused by a _____ in the _____ that aids the process of

_____ excess fluid. The remedy is based on the process of _____. The leaves

should be _____ and not _____ so that it does not interfere with this process.

Most women prefer the leaves to be cooled in the refrigerator as a _____ measure. The leaves should be

placed inside the brassiere, left until _____ and then replaced with _____ leaves. Repeat the process until

_____ is obtained.

PHARMACOLOGY ISSUES IN CHILDBIRTH

 Completion

The following activities relate to pharmacology and childbirth.

5. Complete the following statements.

a. Organogenesis occurs between approximately____ and _____ days post-conception (i.e. ____ and ____ weeks of pregnancy).

b. 'Teratogen' refers to a substance (if it is present in the body during organogenesis) that leads to the birth

of a _____ baby.

c. Factors influencing passage of drugs across the placenta and breast are: i. the _____ of the molecule, ii.

the _____ of the molecule (i.e. +ve or −ve), iii. the lipid or water _____

and iv. the _____ binding capacity. In general, molecules of a _____ size do not cross

the placenta and _____ sized molecules cross very easily.

6. Table 16.3 presents the he physiological changes of pregnancy and how these may influence the way the mother's body handles drugs administered. Complete the table by removing the incorrect word(s).

Table 16.3

	Physiological changes	**Possible effects**
a.	**Prolonged/accelerated** time in the gut	Changes in the **absorption/excretion** of oral drugs
b.	**Increased/decreased** circulating plasma volume results in **increased/decreased** volume	**Increase/decrease** in the plasma concentration
c.	**Increase/decrease** in blood flow to the kidneys	**Increase/decrease** in the rate of excretion of the drug
d.	**Increased/decreased** amounts of total body water and fat	May alter the **distribution/secretion** of the drug
e.	Some metabolic pathways in the liver **increase/decrease**	**Slower/quicker** metabolism
f.	**Major/minor** changes in levels of plasma proteins to which some drugs bind	The amount of drug available is **affected/unaffected**

Possible adverse effects on the fetus

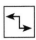 **Matching and completion**

7. Table 16.4 lists drugs that can adversely affect the fetus. Match these correctly to the possible abnormalities (i–v).

i. Reduced fetal growth
ii. Fetal renal failure
iii. Fetal thyroid function
iv. Folate metabolism interference
v. Premature closure of ductus arteriosus and oligohydramnios

Table 16.4

	Drugs
a.	ß-blockers (before 28 weeks):
b.	Angiotensin-converting enzyme (ACE) inhibitors in 2nd and 3rd trimester:
c.	Iodine:
d.	Non-steroidal anti-inflammatory drugs (NSAIDS) in 3rd trimester (e.g. ibuprofen and diclofenac):
e.	Commonly used antibiotic, trimethoprim, in 1st trimester:

8. Table 16.5 shows commonly used drugs that are teratogens. Complete the table by inserting the correct effects from the list provided.

Cardiac defects
Craniofacial, cardiac and CNS abnormalities
Neural tube defects
Craniofacial abnormalities
Facial anomalies, CNS anomalies

Table 16.5

	Commonly used drugs that are teratogens	
	Drug	Effect
a.	Lithium	
b.	Warfarin	
c.	Sodium Valproate	
d.	Phenytoin	
e.	Retinoic acid derivatives	

9. Table 16.6 shows the antibiotics that can cause adverse effects in pregnancy. Complete the table by matching the risks to the correct antibiotic group (i–v).

i. Aminoglycosides (gentamicin, netilmicin)
ii. Chloramphenicol
iii. Nitrofurantoin
iv. Quinolones (ciproflaxin, ofloxacin)
v. Tetracyclines (tetracycline, oxytetracycline, doxycycline)

Table 16.6

	Antibiotics that can cause adverse effects in pregnancy	
	Risk	Antibiotic group (examples)
a.	Discolouration and dysplasia of fetal bones and teeth when used in 2nd and 3rd trimester.	
b.	Risk of ototoxicity but often used in severe maternal infection.	
c.	'Grey baby syndrome' when used in 2nd and 3rd trimester	
d.	Haemolysis in fetus at term – avoid during labour and birth.	
e.	Arthropathy in fetus.	

Miscellaneous

 True/false

10. Table 16.7 provides statements related to drugs in pregnancy and childbirth. Complete the table by deciding if the statements are true or false by ticking the appropriate column.

Table 16.7

	Statement	True	False
a.	Modern antacids are safe for use during pregnancy because they are relatively non-absorbable.		
b.	Hydralazine is usually administered intramuscularly.		
c.	A mother taking a largely fat-soluble drug will pass more to the baby who feeds for prolonged periods (due to the amount of hindmilk consumed).		
d.	Oxytocin should not be given within at least 3–6 hours of prostaglandin because of the risk of uterine hyperstimulation.		
e.	Heparin crosses the placenta and is excreted into breastmilk.		
f.	Paracetamol is the recommended first-line analgesic agent in pregnancy.		
g.	In women with long-term use of opiate analgesics there is no risk of neonatal withdrawal after birth.		
h.	Warfarin is safe in breastfeeding.		
i.	Corticosteroids are used in pregnancy for fetal lung maturation.		

? Multiple choice questions (MCQs)

11. The recommended daily dose of folic acid for all women planning a pregnancy and throughout the first trimester is:

    a. 400 mg   b. 500 mg   c. 400 µg   d. 500 µg

12. Women at risk of neural tube defects should receive a daily dose of folic acid supplementation of:

    a. 2 mg   b. 5 mg   c. 7 mg   d. 10 mg

13. The risk of 'fetal warfarin syndrome' for those exposed is around:

    a. 2%   b. 4%   c. 6%   d. 10%

14. Which of the following drugs affects milk production and would be contraindicated for breastfeeding mothers?

    a. Bromocriptine

    b. Beta blockers

    c. NSAIDS

    d. Methyldopa

17 The baby at birth

This chapter focuses on the baby at birth and their ability to adapt to extrauterine life. As the key professional, the midwife must have sound knowledge of the physiological processes taking place at this time and know how to support the baby through this profound transition phase. The activities will test your knowledge in this area.

Uterine hypoxia

 Completion

1. The following activity relates to the fetal response to intrauterine hypoxia. Complete the activity by inserting the correct word(s) from the list provided.

accelerating	gasping	metabolic acidosis
anaerobic glycolysis	glycogen reserves	oxygen
aspiration	meconium	relaxes
bradycardia	meconium-stained	vessels

The fetus responds to hypoxia by _____ the heart rate in an effort to maintain

supplies of _____ to the brain. If hypoxia persists, glucose depletion will stimulate

_____. This results in a _____. Cerebral _____ will

dilate and some brain swelling may occur. _____ develops as the fetus becomes more acidotic and

cardiac _____ are depleted. The anal sphincter _____ and the fetus

may pass _____ into the liquor. Hypoxia triggers _____, breathing movements which

may result in the _____ of _____ liquor into the lungs.

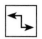 Matching and labelling

2. Figure 17.1 shows the factors predisposing to intrauterine hypoxia. This relates to maternal, fetal or placental issues. Label the figure by matching them with the correct label from the list provided.

Cord prolapse or compression, true knot in cord
Maternal hypertension and vascular disease
Placental disease, dysfunction or separation
Fetal anaemia
Maternal hypoxia, cardiopulmonary disease
Poor perfusion of placental site

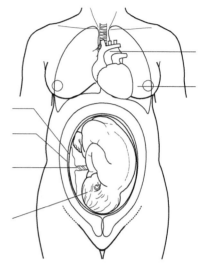

Figure 17.1

Initial assessment of the newborn

Completion

3. The Apgar score is an initial assessment of the baby's condition at birth. The midwife assesses the baby at 1 minute and 5 minutes after birth. Table 17.1 shows the signs and possible scores. Complete the table by inserting the missing word(s) and numerical values.

Table 17.1

Sign	Score		
	0	**1**	**2**
Heart rate	Absent	< ____ bpm	> ____ bpm
Respiratory effort	_____	slow _____ ,	Good or _____
Muscle tone	_____	Some flexion of limbs	_____
Reflex response to stimuli	None	_____	Cough or sneeze
Colour	_____ , _____	_____	_____

4. Complete the following mnemonic for the Apgar score (and the sign it relates to on the APGAR scoring checklist).

A: _____ (relates to _____).

P: _____ (relates to heart rate).

G: Grimace (relates to _____).

A: _____ (relates to _____).

R: _____ (relates to breathing).

Adaptation to extrauterine life

 Completion

5. The following activities relate to the healthy term baby's pulmonary and cardiovascular adaptation to extrauterine life. The activities should be completed by removing the incorrect word(s) and completing the statements as noted.

a. Pulmonary adaptation:

Respiration is stimulated by mild **hypercapnia/hypocapnia**, hypoxia and **alkalosis/acidosis**. There is a change in the rhythm of respiration from **episodic/regular, shallow/deeper** fetal respiration to **episodic/regular, shallow/deeper** breathing. This is due to a combination of chemical and neural stimuli, notably a **fall/rise** in pH level, a **fall/rise** in PaO_2 and a **fall/rise** in $PaCO_2$. Considerable **negative/positive** intrathoracic pressure of up to 9.8 kPa (**50 cm/100 cm** water) is exerted as the first breath is taken. The pressure exerted to effect **exhalation/inhalation increases/diminishes** with each breath taken until only **5 cm/30 cm** of water is required to **deflate/inflate** each lung. This is due to surfactant.

b. List other respiratory stimuli: _____, _____, _____ and pain.

c. Surfactant is a complex of **proteins** and **lipoproteins/carbohydrate substrates**. In utero, the amount of surfactant **decreases/increases** until the lungs are mature at **30–34 weeks'/26–30 weeks'** gestation. It is produced by **type 2/type 1** epithelial cells in the lungs and lines the **alveoli/trachea** to **increase/reduce** the **surface tension/surface area** within the **alveoli/trachea**. This permits **dead air space/residual air** to remain in the **alveoli/trachea** between breaths and prevent them from **deflating/collapsing** at the **beginning/end** of each expiration. Surfactant **increases/reduces** the work or effort of breathing.

d. Cardiovascular adaptation:

At birth, the lungs expand and pulmonary vascular resistance is **lowered/raised**. This results in the majority of cardiac output being sent to the lungs.

Deoxygenated/oxygenated blood returning to the heart from the lungs **increases/decreases** the pressure within the **right/left** atrium. At the same time, pressure in the **right/left** atrium is **raised/lowered** because blood ceases to flow through the cord. This brings about functional closure of the **foramen ovale/ductus venosus**.

Contraction of the walls of the **ductus venosus/ductus arteriosus** occurs almost immediately after birth. This is thought to occur because of the sensitivity of the muscle of the **ductus venosus/ductus arteriosus** to **decreased/increased** oxygen tension and **increased/reduction** in circulating prostaglandins. There is usually functional closure of the **ductus venosus/ductus arteriosus** within **8–10 hours/24–36 hours** of birth with complete closure taking place within **several months/12 months**.

The remaining temporary structures of the fetal circulation – **umbilical vein/ umbilical veins, ductus venosus/ducutus arteriosus** and hypogastric **arteries/veins** – close functionally within a few **minutes/hours** after birth and constriction of the cord. Anatomical closure of fibrous tissue occurs within **2–3 months/12 months**.

Thermal adaptation

6. Complete the following statements in relation to thermal adaptation.

a. Intrauterine temperature is: _____ °C

b. Birthing room temperature is: _____ °C

c. The baby will lose heat in the following ways:

   i. _____ of amniotic fluid from the skin.

   ii. _____ when the baby is in close contact with cold surfaces.

   iii. _____ to cold objects.

   iv. _____ caused by currents of cool air passing over the surface of body.

d. The baby's _____ surface area: body mass ratio potentiates heat loss, especially from the large

   _____.

e. The subcutaneous tissue is _____.

f. The baby has limited ability to _____.

g. The baby is unable to increase _____ voluntarily in order to generate heat.

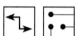 **Matching and labelling**

7. Figure 17.2 shows the modes of heat loss in the neonate. Complete the figure by correctly inserting the following labels:

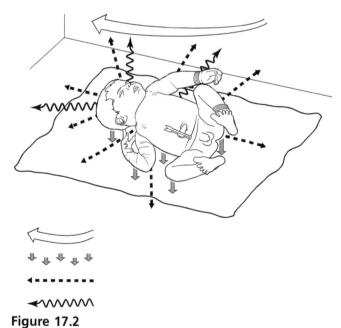

Radiation
Conduction
Evaporation
Convection

Figure 17.2

Colouring

8. Complete Figure 17.3 colouring in all the sites of brown fat in the neonate.

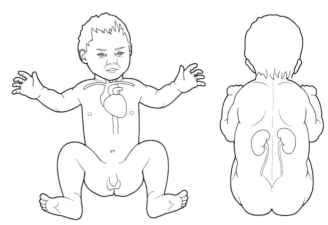

Figure 17.3 Sites of brown fat.

 Completion

9. This activity relates to cold stress and transient tachypnoea of the newborn. Complete the activity by inserting the missing word(s) from the list provided.

acidosis   increases   respiratory rate   tachypnoea

cyanosed   grunt   rib cage   vasoconstriction

decrease   rapid

Cold stress causes _____, thus reducing pulmonary perfusion. Respiratory

_____ develops as the pH and PaO_2 of the blood _____ and the $PaCO_2$ _____

leading to respiratory distress exhibited by _____. This condition is characterized by _____

respirations of up to 120/min. It is common after a caesarean section. The baby may be _____ but

maintains normal blood gases apart from PaO_2. There is little or no recession of the _____ and

there is minimum, if any, _____ on expiration. The _____ may remain elevated for up to

5 days.

Neonatal resuscitation

 Completion

10. This activity relates to the baby at birth showing no sign of respiratory effort. Complete the flow diagram 17.1 by inserting the missing word(s) or numerical values from the list provided. Word(s) may be used more than once.

aerate   dried   radiant heater   ventilate

airway   head   shoulders   ventilation

assisted ventilation   hypothermia   sustained   40

chest movement   inflation   towel

clock timer   nose and mouth trachea

Flow diagram 17.1: Action taken

a. The baby is _____ quickly. The _____ is started. The _____

is switched on to prevent _____.

The head should be put in the neutral position to maintain the _____ and keep the

_____ straightened. If necessary, a small _____ can be put under the baby's

_____ to cause slight extension of the _____. Review for respiratory effort.

↓

b. If the baby fails to respond then _____ is necessary.

Place a correctly fitting face mask to cover the _____ and ensures a good seal. Use

a 500 mL self-inflating bag to _____ the lungs, deliver five _____ inflation

breaths (each inflation breath should be 2–3 seconds). Review for _____.

If **YES** – this is present: continue to _____ at a rate of _____ respirations per minute

(ventilation breaths).

If **NO** – this is not present: then review the _____ position and re-commence the five

_____ breaths. Move into _____ breaths once _____

has been confirmed.

Outcome: Baby is breathing spontaneously.

✎ **Completion**

11. This activity relates to external cardiac massage. Complete the following statements by inserting the correct numerical values.

a. Chest compressions should be performed if the heart rate is <_____ bpm.

b. The chest is depressed at a rate of _____ – _____ times/min, at a ratio of _____ compressions to _____

ventilation and at a depth of _____–_____ cm of the baby's chest. N.B. For resuscitation guidance – always refer to the most current resuscitation guidelines.

True/false

12. Consider the following statements in Table 17.2. Complete the table by deciding if the statements are correct by ticking the appropriate column.

Table 17.2

	Statement	True	False
a.	Before birth, the fetal lung is full of fluid.		
b.	The closure of the foramen ovale cannot be reversed and re-opened.		
c.	The stimuli for respiration results from normal labour, due partially to the intermittent cessation of maternal perfusion with contractions.		
d.	Non-shivering thermogenesis refers to the process involving brown adipose tissue that assists in the rapid mobilization of heat resources from free fatty acids and glycerol in times of cold stress.		
e.	The two thumbs method of chest compression is haemodynamically more effective.		
f.	Brown fat uses the same amount of oxygen as other tissues.		
g.	During primary apnoea, the circulation and heart rate are maintained.		
h.	The body has a high capacity to store vitamin K.		

? Multiple choice questions (MCQs)

13. During birth the fluid leaves the alveoli of the lungs via the:

    a. Thoracic duct or to the lung capillaries

    b. Alveolar walls into the pulmonary lymphatic vessels

    c. Airway and out of the mouth and nose

    d. b and c only

    e. All of the above

14. During fetal life, the percentage of the cardiac output circulated to the fetal lungs through the pulmonary artery is.

    a. 10%   b. 15%   c. 20%   d. 25%

15. What percentage of the body mass does the head of the newborn comprise?

    a. 10%   b. 15%   c. 20%   d. 25%

16. The newborn has sufficient brown fat to meet minimum heat needs after birth for between:

    a. 12–24 hours   b. 2–4 days   c. 4–6 days   d. 6–7 days

17. Which of the following statements is correct about vitamin K:

    a. It is water-soluble

    b. It can only be absorbed from the intestines in the presence of bile salts

    c. The body has a high capacity to store vitamin K

    d. All of the above

18 The newborn baby

This chapter focuses on a variety of situations relating to the newborn baby. This includes the healthy baby, the ill baby and babies who have experienced birth traumas. The activities will test your knowledge in these areas.

Completion

1. The following activity relates to the normal newborn baby at term. Complete the statements by inserting the correct word(s) or numerical values from the extended list provided.

10	30	40	60	100
13	36.0	37.8	72	110
20	36.5	48	85	160
24	37.3	50	90	180

a. The normal core temperature is generally considered to be between _____ and _____°C.

b. The respiratory rate is between _____ and _____ breaths/min.

c. The heart rate is between _____ and _____ beats per min.

d. The haemoglobin level is between _____ and _____ g/dL, of which _____–_____% is fetal haemoglobin.

e. Meconium is passed within _____ hours of birth and is totally excreted within ____–___ hours.

f. The inborn errors of metabolism and disorders routinely screened for (blood spot test) include: _____

_____, _____ and _____.

Definitions

2. Complete the following definitions related to the classification of babies by weight and gestation

a. Low birthweight (LBW) babies are those weighing below _____ g at birth.

b. Very low birthweight (VLBW) babies are those weighing below _____ g at birth.

c. Extremely low birthweight (ELBW) babies are those who weigh below _____ g at birth.

d. A pre-term baby is one born before completion of the _____ th gestational week, regardless of birthweight.

True/false

3. Table 18.1 presents statements relating to the newborn. Complete the table by deciding if the statements are true or false by ticking the appropriate column.

Table 18.1

	Statement	True	False
a.	Vernix caseosa is a white sticky substance present on the baby's skin at birth and flakes off within the first 7 days.		
b.	At birth, the muscles are complete with subsequent growth occurring by hyperplasia rather than hypertrophy.		
c.	Ortolani's test is carried out for dislocation of the hip.		
d.	The low pH (<5) of the baby's skin creates an 'acid mantle' which protects against infection.		
e.	Epithelial pearls (Epstein's pearls) may be observed in the mouth.		
f.	Vasomotor instability causes the harlequin colour change noted on the skin.		
g.	Moro reflex occurs in response to a sudden stimulus.		

 Matching

4. Table 18.2 describes a range of skin observations the midwife may note on routine examination. Match these correctly to the most likely cause or condition (1–14).

1. Bruising	2. Cyanosis	3. Erythema toxicum	4. Herpes simplex
5. Jaundice	6. Milia	7. Miliaria	8. Pallor
9. Petechiae or purpura rash	10. Plethora	11. Skin rashes	12. Staphylococcal
13. Thrush	14. Umbilical sepsis		

Table 18.2

	Statement relating to skin conditions/causes
a.	A pale, mottled baby is an indication of poor peripheral perfusion: _____.
b.	Babies are usually described as being beetroot red. The colour may indicate an excess of circulating red blood cells: _____.
c.	The mucous membranes are the most reliable indicators of central colour in all babies. This indicates low oxygen saturation levels in the blood: _____.
d.	Early onset of this condition (presenting in the first 24 hours) is abnormal: _____.
e.	These are common but most are benign and self-limiting: _____.
f.	These are white or yellow papules over the cheeks, nose and forehead. These disappear in the first weeks of life: _____.
g.	These are clear vesicles on the face, scalp and perineum, caused by the retention of sweat in unopened sweat glands: _____.
h.	These can occur in neonatal thrombocytopenia: _____.
i.	This can ocur extensively following assisted births: _____.
j.	This rash occurs in 30–70% of babies. It consists of white papules on an erythematous base and is benign: _____.
k.	This is a fungal infection of the mouth and throat. It is common in neonates: _____.
l.	This is a most serious viral infection. It presents as a rash with vesicles or pustules: _____.
m.	This can be caused by a bacterial infection on the base of the cord: _____.
n.	Severe infections of this bacteria makes the skin look as though it has been scalded. It can lead to bullous impetigo: _____.

Warning signs

 Completion

5. Table 18.3 shows the general assessment of warning signs indicating a possible underlying problem in the baby. Complete the table by completing or inserting the missing word(s).

Table 18.3

	General assessment warning signs
a.	Skin appearance: P_____. Central cyanosis. J_____.
b.	A_____ lasting longer than 20 seconds.
c.	Heart rate < _____ bpm or > _____ bpm (taken during spells of inactivity).
d.	Respiratory rate < _____ or >_____ breaths per min.
e.	Skin temperature (axilla) <_____ °C or >_____ °C.
f.	Lack of spontaneous movement and _____.
g.	Abnormal lying position either _____ or _____.
h.	Lack of _____ in surroundings.

6. Table 18.4 presents statements of the warning signs of congenital cardiac disease. Complete the table by inserting the correct word(s) from the list provided.

breathless	eyelids	scrotum	tachypnoea
cardiac	feet	sweaty	
cyanosis	gain	systolic	
liver	oedema	tachycardia	

Table 18.4

	Statements
a.	_____ (this is often out of proportion to the degree of respiratory distress)
b.	Persistent _____.
c.	Persistent _____ at rest.
d.	Poor feeding: infants may be _____ and _____ during feeds.
e.	A sudden _____ in weight leading to clinical signs of _____: this is usually noted in the baby having puffy _____ or _____ and in males, the _____ may be swollen.
f.	A very loud _____ murmur is invariably significant.
g.	Evidence of _____ enlargement on X-ray, persisting beyond 48 hours of life.
h.	Enlargement of the _____.

Neonatal problems and conditions

 True/false

7. Table 18.5 presents statements relating to the newborn. Complete the table by deciding if the statements are true or false by ticking the appropriate column.

Table 18.5

	Statement	True	False
a.	Necrotizing enterocolitis (NEC) is an acquired disease of the small and large intestine caused by ischaemia of the intestinal mucosa.		
b.	Hypothermia is defined as a core temperature below 35.5°C.		
c.	Hirschsprung's disease should be suspected in term babies with delayed passage of meconium.		
d.	Respiratory distress syndrome occurs as a result of the insufficient production of surfactant.		
e.	The term hypotonia describes the loss of body tension and tone.		
f.	Hyperthermia is defined as a core temperature above 38.5°C.		
g.	Pre-term infants below 30 weeks' gestation have a resting position that is usually characterised as hypertonic.		
h.	Posseting occurs with winding and overhandling of the baby after feeding.		
i.	At 36–38 weeks' gestation, the resting position of a healthy newborn is one of total flexion with immediate recoil.		

Matching

8. Table 18.6 presents statements related to the signs of respiratory compromise. Complete the table by correctly matching the statements to the relevant terminology.

i. Apnoea   ii. Asynchrony   iii. Grunting

iv. Nasal flaring   v. Retractions   vi. Tachypnoea

Table 18.6

	Statement
a.	The breathing has a see-saw pattern as the abdominal movements and the diaphragm work out of unison: _____.
b.	This is an audible noise heard on expiration: _____.
c.	This occurs with the nares when the body tries to attempt to minimize the effect of the airways resistance by maximizing the diameter of the upper airways: _____.
d.	Chest distortions occur due to an increase in the need to create higher respiratory pressures in a compliant chest. They appear across the thorax: _____.
e.	This is a compensatory rise in the respiratory rate initiated by the respiratory centre. The rise aims to remove hypercarbia and prevent hypoxia: _____.
f.	This is the absence of breathing for more than 20 seconds: _____.

Definition

9. Complete the following definition by inserting the missing word(s).

A neutral thermal environment is defined as the _____ air temperature at which

_____ consumption or _____ production is _____, with body

temperature in the normal range.

The remainder of the main activities relates to birth traumas.

Caput succedaneum and cephalhaematoma

 Short answers

10. Complete the following short answers.

a. Caput succedaneum

What does this term refer to? _____

_____

When does it occur? _____

_____

What causes this condition: _____

_____

b. Cephalhaematoma

What does this term refer to? _____

_____

When does it occur? _____

_____

What causes this condition: _____

_____

_____

  Colour and labelling

11. Figure 18.1 shows a caput succedaneum. Colour and label as noted.

Label

Skull
Periosteum
Scalp

Colour and label

Blood and serum

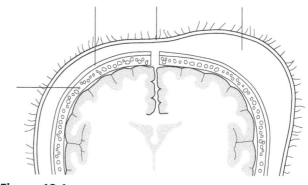

Figure 18.1

12. Figure 18.2 shows a cephalhaematoma. Colour and label as noted.

Label

skull
periosteum
scalp

Colour and label

Blood

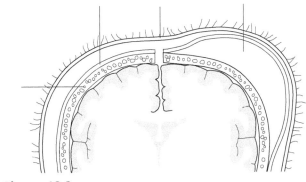

Figure 18.2

 Matching

13. Table 18.7 presents a list of statements. Complete the table by ticking the relevant box to indicate if each statement relates to caput succedaneum or cephalhaematoma.

Table 18.7

	Statement	Cephalhaematoma	Caput succudaneum
a.	It is not present at birth.		
b.	It does not enlarge.		
c.	The swelling feels firm.		
d.	It is present at birth.		
e.	It can cross a suture line.		
f.	The swelling may move.		
g.	It may be bilateral.		
h.	The swelling appears after 12 hours.		
i.	It can 'pit' on pressure.		
j.	It may result in hyperbilirubinaemia.		
k.	The swelling grows larger over days.		
l.	It is resolved by 36 hours after birth.		
m.	It can persist for weeks.		
n.	A 'false' swelling can also occur with a vacuum extraction.		
o.	It subsides when the blood is reabsorbed.		
p.	It does not 'pit' on pressure.		
q.	It does not cross a suture line.		
r.	A ridge of bone may be felt around the edge of the swelling.		
s.	The swelling is fixed.		

Birth Injuries

14. Table 18.8 presents statements relating to birth injuries. Consider these and match correctly to the injury (1–9).

1. Brachial plexus

4. Skin damage

7. Subarachnoid haemorrhage

2. Erb's palsy

5. Total brachial palsy

8. Torticollis

3. Klumpe's palsy

6. Subdural haemorrhage

9. Umbilical haemorrhage

Table 18.8

	Statement
a.	Damage to this organ is often iatrogenic, resulting from instrumental births: _____.
b.	Damage is caused by excessive traction or twisting causing tearing to muscle(s) during the birth of the anterior shoulder or rotation of shoulders in a breech or C/S. The most common is the sternomastoid muscle: _____.
c.	i. This trauma results from excessive lateral flexion, rotation or traction of the head and neck during vaginal breech or shoulder dystocia: _____. ii. The three main types of this nerve injury include: _____, _____, _____.
d.	This injury may occur to the fetal head if excessive compression or abnormal stretching tears the tentorium cerebella: _____.
e.	Pre-term babies who suffer hypoxia resulting in disruption of cerebral blood flow may suffer from this injury: _____.
f.	This results from poorly applied cord ligature: _____.

? Pot luck multiple choice questions (MCQs)

15. Weight loss is normal in the first few days but is deemed to be abnormal if the weight loss is more than:

  a. 2%   b. 5%   c. 10%   d. 15%

16. The Moro reflex is present in the newborn for the first:

  a. 4 weeks   b. 6 weeks   c. 8 weeks   d. 10 weeks

17. Pseudomenstruation in the first days of life is due to the withdrawal of:

  a. Progesterone

  b. Oestrogen

  c. Relaxin

  d. All of the above

18. During a convulsion the baby may have:

  a. Tachycardia

  b. Hypertension

  c. Raised cerebral blood flow

  d. Raised intracranial pressure

  e. a and d

  f. All of the above

19. The percentage of all births affected with a cardiac defect is:

  a. 1%   b. 3%   c. 5%   d. 7%

20. In relation to newborn, management of blood glucose levels keeps levels above the lowest level of normal which is:

  a. 2.4 mmol/dL

  b. 2.6 mmol/dL

  c. 2.8 mmol/dL

  d. 3.0 mmol/dL

CHAPTER
19 Jaundice and blood group incompatibility

The main focus of this chapter is jaundice and blood group incompatibility. These are areas that midwives deal with on a regular basis and a sound knowledge is required. The activities will test your knowledge in these areas.

JAUNDICE

Physiological jaundice

 Completion

1. Conjugation changes the end-products of red cell breakdown so they can be excreted in faeces or urine. Haemoglobin from these cells is broken down to the by-products of haem, globin and iron. Complete the following related statements using the list provided.

amino acids	bilirubin	new	red cells
biliverdin	body	proteins	unconjugated

   a. Haem is converted to _____ and then to _____ _____.

   b. Globin is broken down into _____ and used by the body to make _____.

   c. Iron is stored in the _____ or used for _____ _____.

2. The following activity relates to the two main forms of bilirubin in the body. Complete the two sentences by removing the incorrect word(s) so that these read correctly.

   a. **Unconjugated/conjugated** bilirubin is **fat soluble/water soluble** and cannot be excreted easily in bile or urine.

   b. **Unconjugated/conjugated** bilirubin has been made **fat soluble/water soluble** in the liver and can be excreted in faeces and urine.

3. The following activity in Flow diagram 19.1 (i–iii) breaks down the three stages involved in the process of bilirubin conjugation, i.e. transport, conjugation and excretion. Complete each stage by inserting the correct word(s) from the list provided. A few word(s) may be used more than once.

albumin	enzyme	nerve	urobilinogen
bacteria	faeces	oxygen	urine
biliary	fat soluble	toxicity	
bilirubin	fatty	water-soluble	
brain	glucose	urobilin	

Flow diagram 19.1

i.   Transport of bilirubin:

Unconjugated or _____ bilirubin is transported to the liver bound to

_____. If not attached to _____ then this unbound or 'free'

_____ can be deposited in extravascular _____ and _____ tissues (skin

and _____). Skin deposits of unconjugated or _____ bilirubin cause jaundice,

while _____ deposits can cause 'bilirubin _____' or kernicterus.

↓

ii. Conjugation:

Once in the liver, unconjugated bilirubin is detached from _____, combined

with _____ and glucoronic acid and conjugation occurs in the presence of

_____ and the _____ uridine diphosphoglucuronyl transferase

(UDP-GT). The conjugated bilirubin is now _____ and available for excretion.

↓

iii. Excretion:

Conjugated bilirubin is excreted via the _____ system into the small intestine where normal

_____ change the conjugated bilirubin into _____. This is then

oxidized into orange-coloured _____. Most is excreted in the _____ with a

small amount excreted in the _____.

Neonatal physiological jaundice

Completion

4. Complete the following statements relating to neonatal physiological jaundice by inserting the correct word(s).

Neonatal physiological jaundice occurs when unconjugated (_____ soluble) bilirubin is deposited

in the _____ instead of being taken to the _____ for processing into conjugated

(_____ soluble) bilirubin that can be excreted in _____ or _____. It is a normal

transitional state affecting up to _____ % of term babies and _____% of preterm babies who have a

progressive rise in _____ bilrubin levels with jaundice on day _____.

Physiological jaundice **never** appears before _____ hours of life and usually fades by _____ week and bilirubin

levels never exceed _____ – _____ µmol/L (_____ – ___ mg/dL).

Matching

5. Table 19.1 presents straightforward statements that relate to the causes of neonatal physiological jaundice. Match the statements correctly to the possible cause (i–iv).

i. Enzyme deficiency

ii. Decreased albumin-binding capacity

iii. Increased enterohepatic reabsorption

iv. Increased red cell breakdown

Table 19.1

	Statement
a.	Newborns have lower concentrations and the decrease in capacity reduces the transport of bilirubin to the liver. _____
b.	When the baby is born and the pulmonary system becomes functional then there is haemolysis of the large cell mass no longer required. This results in an increased level of unconjugated bilirubin. _____
c.	Drugs also compete for these sites and this leaves less capacity for bilirubin transport. _____
d.	If all sites are used then levels of unbound 'free' fat soluble bilirubin rises in the blood and finds tissues with the affinity for fat. _____
e.	The newborn bowel lacks the normal enteric bacteria that breaks down conjugated bilirubin to urobilinogen. _____
f.	Levels of activity are lower during the first 24 hours after birth and this reduces the conjugation of bilirubin in the liver. _____

Pathological neonatal jaundice

 Short answers

6. Complete the following activities referring to the textbook as required.

a. Kernicterus (bilirubin toxicity) is an _____pathy caused by _____ of _____ bilirubin in the _____ ganglia of the _____.

b. Early signs can be _____ and include (identify at least two): _____

_____

_____

c. Long-term clinical features can include (identify at least four): _____

_____

_____

_____

7. Complete the following statements related to the criteria for diagnosis of pathological jaundice of the newborn by inserting the correct numerical values from the list provided.

1.5	5	12.0	35
2.0	7	24	85
2	10	25	200

   a.   Pathological jaundice usually occurs within the first _____ hours of life.

   b.   A rapid increase in total serum bilirubin >_____ μmol/L (_____ mg/dL) per day.

   c.   Total serum bilirubin >_____ μmol/L (_____ m/dL).

   d.   Conjugated bilirubin >_____ – _____ μmol/L (_____ – _____ mg/dL)

   e.   Persistence of jaundice for ___ – _____ days or ____ weeks in pre-term babies.

Matching

8. Table 19.2 presents statements relating to the neonate and the interference in bilirubin production, transport, conjugation and excretion which causes pathological jaundice (1–4). Consider these statements and complete the table by matching them to the relevant cause.

1. Conjugation   2. Excretion

3. Production   4. Transport

Table 19.2

	Statement
a.	Blood type/group incompatibility. _____
b.	Immaturity of the enzyme system. _____
c.	Drugs that compete with bilirubin for albumin-binding sites. _____
d.	Hepatic obstruction. _____
e.	Spherocytosis. _____
f.	Infection, idiopathic neonatal hepatitis. _____ and ____ _____
g.	Acidosis, hypothermia or hypoxia. _____
h.	Obstruction by 'bile plugs' (e.g. cystic fibrosis). _____
i.	Polycythemia. _____
j.	Extravasated blood (cephalhaematoma or bruising). _____
k.	Metabolic or endocrine disorders that alter UDP-GT enzyme activity. _____

BLOOD GROUP INCOMPATIBILITY

 Completion

9. The following activity relates to the causes of haemolytic jaundice through maternal blood group types. Complete the following two paragraphs by removing the incorrect word so that they read correctly.

a. RhD **incompatibility/compatibility** can occur when a woman with **Rh-negative/Rh-positive** blood type is pregnant with a **Rh-negative/Rh-positive fetus**. The placenta acts as a barrier to fetal blood entering the maternal circulation. During pregnancy or birth, fetomaternal haemorrhage (FMH) can occur when small amounts of fetal **Rh-negative/Rh-positive** blood cross the placenta and enter the **Rh-positive/Rh-negative** mother's blood. The woman's immune system produces **anti-D/anti-O** antibodies. In subsequent pregnancies these maternal antibodies can cross the placenta and destroy the red cells of any **Rh-negative/Rh-positive** fetus.

b. ABO **isoimmunization/immunization** usually occurs when the mother is blood **group O/group A** and the baby is blood **group A/group O** (or less often **group AB/group B**). Individuals with **type O/type A** blood develop antibodies throughout life from exposure to antigens in food, Gram-**negative/positive** bacteria or blood transfusion. The woman usually has high serum **anti-A/anti AO** and **anti AO/anti-B** antibody titres by the time she is pregnant for the first time. Some women produce **IgA/IgG** antibodies that can cross the placenta and attach to the red cells and destroy them.

Miscellaneous

 True/false

10. Consider the statements presented in Table 19.3. Decide if these are true or false by ticking the appropriate column.

Table 19.3

	Statement	True	False
a.	Mothers should be advised to continue to breastfeed if the baby experiences prolonged jaundice.		
b.	Pre-term babies are at risk of physiological jaundice because the shorter red cell life increases production of unconjugated bilirubin.		
c.	Anti-D antibodies are the most common type.		
d.	ABO incompatibility is the most frequent cause of mild-moderate haemolysis in the neonate.		
e.	In relation to Rhesus factor inheritance: the baby will always have Rhesus positive blood group if born to a Rhesus negative (dd) mother and a Rhesus positive (DD homozygous) father		
f.	In neonatal meningitis, very early signs may be non-specific and then followed by meningeal irritation, signs of raised intracranial pressure and alterations to consciousness.		
g.	Toxoplasmosis is a protozoan parasite found in uncooked meat and cat and dog faeces.		

20 Congenital abnormalities and metabolic disorders

This chapter is focused on congenital abnormalities and metabolic disorders. The midwife is often the first to notice an abnormality in a baby either during the birth process or in the early postnatal period. It is essential to have knowledge of these conditions to provide appropriate care to the baby and support the parents. The activities will test your knowledge of the main abnormalities and disorders.

Inherited disorders

A congenital abnormality is any defect in form, structure or function.

 True/false

1. Table 20.1 presents statements relating to inherited disorders. Consider each statement and decide whether they are true or false by ticking the appropriate column.

Table 20.1

	Statements	True	False
a.	A recessive gene needs to be present on both chromosomes before producing its effect.		
b.	Mitosis is cell division that occurs in somatic cells where each new cell gets a full set of chromosomes.		
c.	The zygote should have one sex chromosome and 23 autosomes from each parent.		
d.	Mitochondria are always inherited from the father.		
e.	Meiosis is the type of cell reduction that occurs in the formation of gametes, in which one of each chromosome pair is lost.		
f.	A dominant gene will produce its effect even if present in only one chromosome of a pair.		
g.	Trisomy refers to a situation where a particular chromosome is represented three times in the nucleus.		
h.	In an X-linked recessive inheritance the condition affects almost exclusively females, although males can be carriers.		
i.	Cystic fibrosis is an autosomal recessive condition.		
j.	Duchenne muscular dystrophy is an example of an X-linked recessive inheritance.		
k.	Trisomy 21 is an example of a chromosomal abnormality.		
l.	Haemophilia is an example of an X-linked dominant inheritance.		
m.	Turner's syndrome is an example of a monosomal condition where there is only one sex chromosome.		

Congenital defects and conditions

  Matching and completion

2. Table 20.2 presents statements about defects and conditions. Consider these statements and then match to the condition in the list provided (1–13).

1. Choanal atresia
2. Cleft lip and palate
3. Diaphragmatic hernia
4. Exomphalos
5. Gastroschisis
6. Hirschsprung's disease
7. Imperforate anus
8. Malrotation/volvulus
9. Meconium ileus (cystic fibrosis)
10. Oesophageal atresia
11. Pierre Robin sequence
12. Pyloric stenosis
13. Rectal atresia

Table 20.2

	Statement
a.	One characteristic of this condition is micrognathia (hypoplasia of the lower jaw): _____
b.	There is an aganglionic section of the bowel: _____
c.	This condition arises from a genetic defect that causes hypertrophy of the muscles of the pyloric sphincter: _____
d.	There is herniation of the abdominal contents into the thoracic cavity: _____
e.	These five conditions may be suspected if the baby fails to pass meconium in the first 24 hours after birth: _____ , _____ , _____ , _____ , _____ .
f.	This defect may be unilateral or bilateral. It may affect the soft palate, hard palate or both: _____
g.	This is a defect where the bowel or other viscera protrude through the umbilicus: _____
h.	This is a unilateral or bilateral narrowing of the nasal passages with a web of tissue or bone occluding the nasopharynx: _____
i.	In this condition there is incomplete canalization of the oesophagus in early uterine development: _____
j.	This is a paramedian defect of the abdominal wall with extrusion of bowel that is not covered with peritoneum: _____

Cardiac defects

 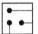 **Colouring, labelling and completion**

3. Figure 20.1 shows the normal heart. Label as indicated. Colour the flow of oxygenated and deoxygenated blood through the normal heart (refer to a coloured physiology textbook to check your response).

Label

Aorta
Right atrium
Left atrium
Pulmonary artery
Right ventricle
Left ventricle

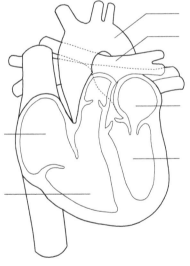

Colour and identify the direction of flow

Flow of blood through the aorta

Flow of blood through the pulmonary artery

Figure 20.1

4. Complete the statement (i–iii) about the description of the transposition of the great arteries by removing the incorrect word(s) so that the statements read correctly.

   i.   In this condition the aorta arises from the **right/left** ventricle and the pulmonary artery arises from the **left/right** ventricle.

   ii. **Oxygenated/deoxygenated** blood is circulated back through the lungs and **oxygenated/deoxygenated** blood is circulated back into the systemic circulation.

   iii. A **patent ductus venosus/ductus arteriosus** needs to be maintained to provide opportunity for **oxygenated/deoxygenated** blood to access the systemic circulation. Otherwise the baby will die.

5. Figure 20.2 shows tetralogy of Fallot (VSD – ventricular septal defect). Compare with the normal heart structure in Figure 20.1 (A) to highlight the defects. Colour and label as noted (refer to a coloured physiology textbook to check your response).

Label

Aorta
Subpulmonary stenosis
Pulmonary artery
Right ventricular hypertrophy
Ventricular septal defect
(VSD)

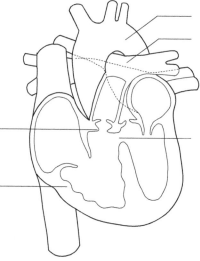

Colour

Oxygenated blood flow
through vessels
Deoxygenated blood flow
through vessels

Figure 20.2

6. Complete the statement about tetralogy of Fallot defect by inserting the missing word(s).

   In this condition there are four key cardiac defects. These include the following:

   i.   pulmonary outflow is _____

   ii. ventricular septal defect (VSD)

   iii. right ventricle is _____

   iv. an _____ aorta

7. There are a small number of cardiac defects that may not require medical/surgical treatment in early life. These will require careful follow-up of signs of developing heart failure at a later stage and may then require treatment. List three cardiac defects within this category:

   i.   _____

   ii. _____

   iii. _____

Short answers

8. Detailed examination of the newborn will reveal the following subtle signs of cardiac failure in situations involving ventricular septal defects. Complete the following statements.

   a. There will be increased respiration rate. This is known as _____.

   b. There will be increased heart rate. This is known as _____.

   c. There will be incipient _____ especially following exertion of crying or feeding.

   d. On auscultation _____ _____ may be heard.

Spina bifida

 Definitions

9. Complete the following definitions related to spina bifida.

    a. Spina bifida results from _____ of fusion of the _____ _____.

    b. A meningocele refers to the protrusion of the _____ through the defect. It does _____

       contain _____ tissue.

    c. Meningomyocele refers to the protrusion of _____ through the defect and it involves

       the _____ _____.

    d. Encephalocele is the term used when the defect is at the _____ of the _____ of the skull.

 Colouring and labelling

10. Figure 20.3 shows various forms of spina bifida. Colour and label as noted (refer to a coloured physiology textbook for a detailed answer).

Colour and label on the 'normal' vertebra

Skin
Spinal cord
Dura

Label on the 'normal' vertebra

Vertebral arch
Nerve

Colour on the other four figures

Skin
Spinal cord
Dura

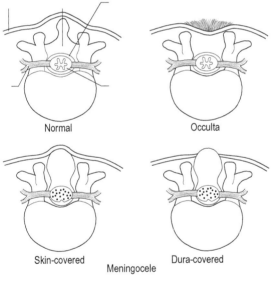

Normal

Occulta

Skin-covered

Dura-covered

Meningocele

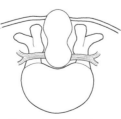

Flat meningomyelocele

Figure 20.3

Miscellaneous congenital defects

 Matching

11. Table 20.3 provides statements relating to a variety of defects. Consider these and correctly match them to the list of congenital defects listed (1–9).

1. Achondroplasia   2. Cryptorchidism   3. Fetal alcohol syndrome/spectrum

4. Hypospadias   5. Osteogenesis imperfecta   6. Port wine stain

7. Potter syndrome   8. Talipes calcaneovalgus   9. Talipes equinovarus

Table 20.3

	Statement
a.	This autosomal dominant disorder of collagen production leads to brittle bones: _____
b.	This is an autosomal dominant condition where the baby is small with a disproportionately large head and short limbs: _____
c.	This is a purple-blue malformation affecting the face. It is fully formed at birth and does not regress with time: _____
d.	The urethral meatus opens onto the under surface of the penis: _____
e.	This refers to undescended testes which may be unilateral or bilateral: _____
f.	The characteristics are a growth-restricted infant with microcephaly, close set eyes, small upturned nose, thin upper lip, close set ears. There are learning difficulties: _____
g.	In this foot deformity the foot is dorsiflexed and everted: _____
h.	The baby's face has a flattened appearance, low set ears, and is incompatable with life because of lung hypoplasia: _____
i.	In this foot deformity the ankle is bent downwards (plantarflexed) and the front part of the foot is turned inwards (inverted): _____

Miscellaneous

 Completion

12. This activity relates to the baby born to a diabetic mother. Complete the paragraph by removing the incorrect words so that it reads correctly.

These infants have **low/high** blood glucose concentrations because of the excess of **insulin/glucogen**. This is produced by the fetal **pancreatic gland/liver** as a result of stimulation by **increased/decreased** maternal **insulin/glucose** concentrations. This excess of **insulin/glucose** also acts as a **growth factor/growth inhibitor** and brings about **reduced/excessive** fat and glycogen deposition. The baby usually has a macrosomic appearance.

True/false

13. Table 20.4 presents statements relating to metabolic and other disorders. Consider the statements and decide if they are true or false by ticking the appropriate column.

Table 20.4

	Statement	True	False
a.	Hypernatraemia in the presence of weight gain suggests dehydration.		
b.	Hypocalcaemia can cause tremors, jitteriness, lethargy and poor feeding.		
c.	Phenylketonuria (PKU) is an autosomal recessive disorder.		
d.	Infants with galactosaemia will test positive for glucose in the urine.		
e.	Thyroid stimulating hormone (TSH) is produced by the posterior pituitary gland.		
f.	Phenylketonuria (PKU) can be treated with a diet specifically restricted in phenylalanine.		
g.	Galactosaemia is a disorder caused by the absence or deficiency of the enzyme galactose-1-phosphate uridyltransferase (Gal-1-P UT).		
h.	Infants with hypothyroidism tend to be large, postmature and have a large posterior fontanelle.		
i.	Opiates cross the placenta and the fetus is likely to be exposed to the same peaks and troughs of drug exposure as the mother.		
j.	Cocaine has harmful effects on the baby including significant fetal growth restriction, brain injury due to haemorrhage or infarction, abnormalities of brain development, limb reduction and gut atresias.		

The female pelvis and pelvic floor

ANSWERS

1. **a.** Ischium   **b.** Sacrum   **c.** Ilium
    d. Sacrum   **e.** Ischium   **f.** Coccyx
    g. Ischium   **h.** Coccyx   **i.** Sacrum
    j. Ilium   **k.** Ischium   **l.** Sacrum
    m. Sacrum   **n.** Ilium   **o.** Sacrum
    p. Sacrum

2.

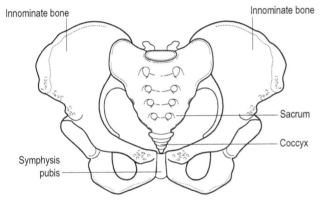

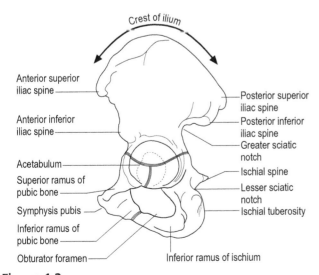

Figure 1.1

3.

Figure 1.2

4. **1.** The symphysis pubis is the midline cartilaginous joint uniting the <u>rami</u> of the <u>left</u> and <u>right pubic bones</u>.

    2. The sacroiliac joints join the <u>sacrum</u> to the <u>ilium</u> and as a result connect the <u>spine</u> to the <u>pelvis</u>.

    3. The sacrococcygeal joint is formed where the <u>base</u> of the <u>coccyx</u> articulates with the <u>tip</u> of the sacrum.

5.

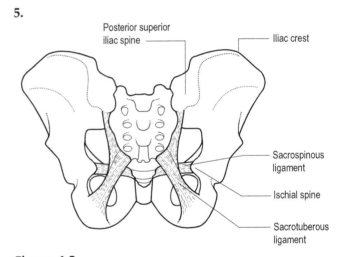

Figure 1.3

6.

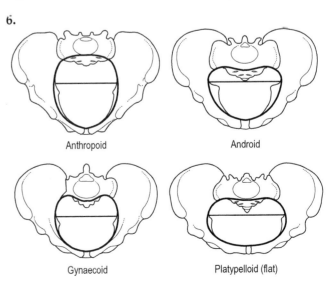

Anthropoid   Android

Gynaecoid   Platypelloid (flat)

Figure 1.4

7.

Table 1.2

Features	Gynaecoid	Anthropoid	Platypelloid	Android
Brim	Rounded	Long oval	Kidney-shaped	Heart-shaped
Forepelvis	Generous	Narrowed	Wide	Narrow
Side walls	Straight	Divergent	Divergent	Convergent

8.

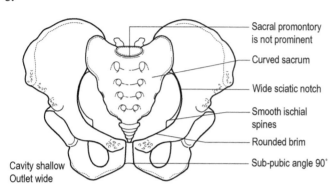

- Sacral promontory is not prominent
- Curved sacrum
- Wide sciatic notch
- Smooth ischial spines
- Rounded brim
- Sub-pubic angle 90°

Cavity shallow
Outlet wide

Figure 1.5

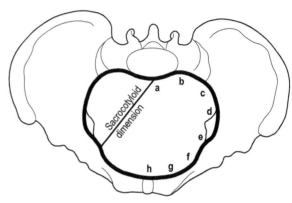

Figure 1.6

9. a. Gynaecoid **b.** Platypelloid **c.** Android
d. Android **e.** Anthropoid **f.** Gynaecoid
g. Android **h.** Platypelloid **i.** Android
j. Android **k.** Gynaecoid **l.** Anthropoid
m. Anthropoid **n.** Android **o.** Anthropoid
p. Platypelloid **q.** Anthropoid, Platypelloid
r. Android **s.** Gynaecoid **t.** Gynaecoid,
Anthropoid, Playpelloid **u.** Android

10. 1. The true pelvis is the <u>bony canal</u> through which the <u>fetus</u> must pass during <u>birth</u>.

2. The true pelvis is divided into three components: **a.** <u>Pelvic brim</u>, **b.** <u>Pelvic cavity</u>, **c.** <u>Pelvic outlet</u>.

3. The false pelvis is the part of the pelvis which is situated <u>above</u> the <u>pelvic brim</u>. It is formed by the <u>upper flared-out</u> portions of the <u>iliac</u> bones and protects the <u>abdominal</u> organs.

11. a. Sacral promontory **b.** Sacral ala or wing **c.** Sacroiliac joint **d.** Iliopectineal line (which is the edge formed at the inward aspect of the ilium) **e.** Iliopectineal eminence (which is the roughened area formed where the superior ramus of the pubic bone meets the ilium) **f.** Superior ramus of the pubic border **g.** Upper inner border of the pubic bone **h.** Upper inner border of the symphysis pubis

12.

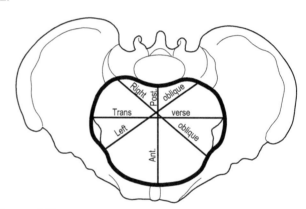

Figure 1.7

13. 1. The transverse diameter extends across the <u>greatest width</u> of the <u>brim</u>.

2. The oblique diameter extends from the <u>iliopectineal eminence</u> of one side to the <u>sacroiliac</u> articulation of the opposite side.

3. The anteroposterior diameter extends from the <u>sacral promontory</u> to the <u>symphysis pubis</u>. The other term for this diameter is the <u>conjugate</u> diameter.

14.

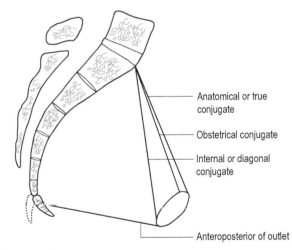

	Anteroposterior	Oblique	Transverse
Brim	11	12	13
Cavity	12	12	12
Outlet	13	12	11

Figure 1.8

15. a. Anatomical conjugate   **b.** Obstetrical conjugate   **c.** Diagonal (Internal) conjugate   **d.** Anatomical conjugate   **e.** Obstetrical conjugate   **f.** Obstetrical conjugate   **g.** Diagonal (Internal) conjugate   **h.** Diagonal (Internal) conjugate   **i.** Obstetrical conjugate   **j.** Anatomical conjugate, obstetrical conjugate

16.

Anatomical or true conjugate

Obstetrical conjugate

Internal or diagonal conjugate

Anteroposterior of outlet

Figure 1.9

17. 1. Engagement may necessitate <u>lateral</u> tilting of the head, known as asynclitism, in order to allow the <u>biparietal</u> diameter to pass the narrowest <u>anteroposterior</u> diameter of the brim.

2. In anterior asynclitism, the <u>anterior</u> parietal bone moves down behind the <u>symphysis pubis</u> until the <u>parietal eminence</u> enters the brim. The movement is then reversed and the head tilts in the <u>opposite</u> direction until the <u>posterior</u> parietal bone negotiates the <u>sacral promontory</u> and the head is engaged.

3. In posterior asynclitism, the movements of anterior asynclitism are <u>reversed</u>. The <u>posterior</u> parietal bone negotiates the <u>sacral promontory</u> prior to the <u>anterior</u> parietal bone moving down behind the <u>symphysis pubis</u>. Once the pelvic brim has been negotiated, <u>descent</u> progresses normally accompanied by <u>flexion</u> and <u>internal</u> rotation.

18. True: b, c, e, i, j, m, p, q

False: a, d, f, g, h, k, l, n, o, r

19. 1. a.   **2.** b.   **3.** a.   **4.** a.   **5.** c.   **6.** a.   **7.** c.   **8.** b.

20. 1. a.   **2.** d.   **3.** d.   **4.** e.

21. 1.   Dietary deficiency

Example 1. Deficiency of vitamins and minerals – rare occurrence.

a.   Rachitic pelvis – this form of pelvis is deformed by rickets in early childhood. It is caused by malnutrition.

b.   The weight of the upper body presses downwards onto softened pelvic bones. The sacral promontory is pushed downwards and forwards. The ischium and ilium are drawn outwards. This results in a flat pelvic brim (similar to the platypelloid pelvis). The sacral is usually straight and the coccyx bends acutely forward. There is a wide pubic arch due to the widened distance between the ischial tuberosities. Bow legs and spinal deformities are signs of rickets.

c.   Caesarean section may be required if severe contraction of the pelvis is evident. The fetal head will attempt to enter the pelvic brim by asynclitism.

Example 2. Osteomalacia pelvis – this form of pelvis is rare in the UK.

a.   It is due to an acquired deficiency of calcium and this condition occurs in adults.

b.   The bones of the skeleton soften due to the gross lack of calcium. The pelvic canal is squashed together until the brim becomes a Y-shaped slit.

c.   Labour is impossible. In early pregnancy the gravid uterus may become incarcerated due to gross deformity.

2.   Developmental anomalies

Example 1: Naegele's pelvis.

a.   It is a rare malformation caused by failure in development.

b. One sacral ala is missing and the sacrum is fused to the ilium causing a grossly asymmetrical pelvic brim.

Example 2: Robert's pelvis.

a. This is a rare malformation caused by failure in development.

b. The malformations are similar to Naegele's pelvis with the deformities being bilateral.

c. In both examples the difficulty is related to engagement of the fetal head due to the abnormal shaped brim.

3. Injury and disease

Example 1: Spinal deformity.

a. If <u>kyphosis</u> (forward angulation) or <u>scoliosis</u> (lateral curvature) is evident or suggested by a limp or deformity, then the woman needs to be referred to a doctor for medical assessment and monitoring.

b. It is usual to have some form of pelvic contraction due to the spinal deformities.

22. **1. a.** It provides support for the pelvic organs.
b. It is important in the maintenance of continence (bladder and bowels) as part of the anal and urinary sphincters. **c.** It has an important role in sexual intercourse.

2. The pelvic floor influences the passive movements of the fetus through the birth canal and relaxes to allow the fetus to exit from the pelvis.

23.

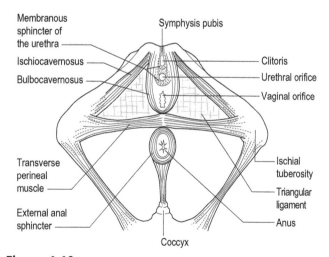

Figure 1.10

24.

Table 1.5

Superficial muscle	Describe the pathway of the muscle(s) and detail any structures of attachment involved
External anal sphincter	Encircles the <u>anus</u> and is attached <u>posteriorly</u> by a few fibres to the <u>coccyx</u>
Ischiocavernosus muscles	Passes from the <u>ischial tuberosities</u> along the <u>pubic arch</u> to the corpora cavernosa
Bulbocavernosus muscles	Passes from the perineum forwards around the <u>vagina</u> to the corpora cavernosa of the <u>clitoris</u> just under the <u>pubic arch</u>
Transverse perineal muscles	Passes from the <u>ischial tuberosities</u> to the centre of the <u>perineum</u>
Membranous sphincter of the urethra	Composed of muscle fibres passing <u>above</u> and <u>below</u> the <u>urethra</u> and attached to the <u>pubic bones</u>

25.

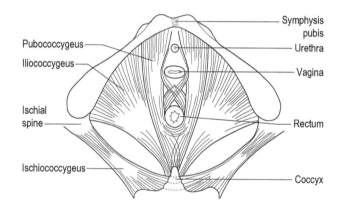

Figure 1.11

26. **a.** Pubococcygeus **b.** Iliococcygeus **c.** Ischiococcygeus **d.** Iliococcygeus **e.** Pubococcygeus, Puborectalis **f.** Iliococcygeus **g.** Iliococcygeus **h.** Puborectalis **i.** Ischiococcygeus

27. True: b, d, g, i, j

False: a, c, e, f, h

The reproductive systems

ANSWERS

1.

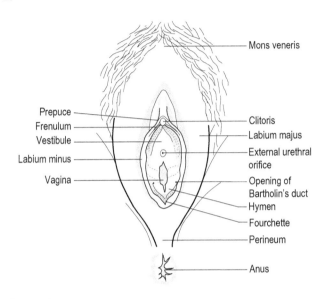

Mons veneris

Prepuce
Frenulum
Vestibule
Labium minus
Vagina

Clitoris
Labium majus
External urethral orifice
Opening of Bartholin's duct
Hymen
Fourchette
Perineum

Anus

Figure 2.1

2. a–ii b–vi c– viii d–i e–vii f–ix g–x
h–iii i–v j–iv

3.

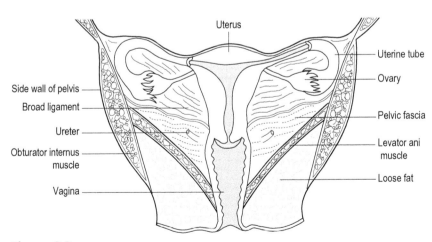

Uterus

Side wall of pelvis
Broad ligament
Ureter
Obturator internus muscle
Vagina

Uterine tube
Ovary
Pelvic fascia
Levator ani muscle
Loose fat

Figure 2.2

4.

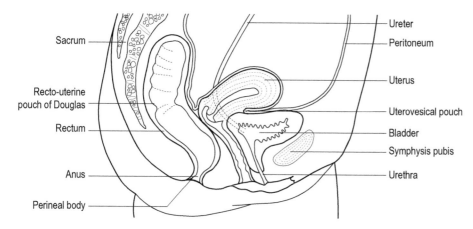

Sacrum

Recto-uterine
pouch of Douglas

Rectum

Anus

Perineal body

Ureter
Peritoneum
Uterus
Uterovesical pouch
Bladder
Symphysis pubis
Urethra

Figure 2.3

5.

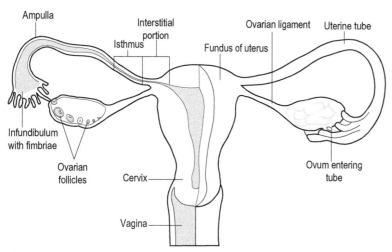

Ampulla

Isthmus

Interstitial
portion

Fundus of uterus

Ovarian ligament   Uterine tube

Infundibulum
with fimbriae

Ovarian
follicles

Cervix

Ovum entering
tube

Vagina

Figure 2.4

6.

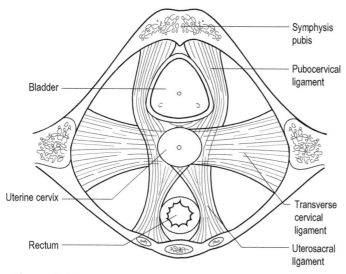

Bladder

Uterine cervix

Rectum

Symphysis
pubis

Pubocervical
ligament

Transverse
cervical
ligament

Uterosacral
ligament

Figure 2.5

7. True – a, c, d, f, g, i, j, k, m, n, p, q

False – b, e, h, l, o

8. The uterus is a hollow **pear**-shaped **muscular** organ located in the **true** pelvis between the **bladder** and the **rectum**. The position of the uterus within the **true** pelvis is one of **ante**-version and **ante**-flexion. **Ante**-version means that the uterus leans **forward** and **ante**-flexion means that it bends forwards upon itself. When the woman is standing, the uterus is in an almost **horizontal** position with the **fundus** resting on the bladder.

9. d.

10. d.

11. a.

12. a. i. 2.5 cm   ii. 10 cm   iii. 7.5 cm

b. i. 7.5 cm   ii. 5 cm   iii. 2.5 cm   iv. 1.25 cm

c. 10 cm

d. pH 4.5

13. Doderlein's bacilli acts on glycogen to form lactic acid.

14. Lesser lips

15. Greater lips

16. Vault

17. a. Mucosa   **b.** Muscle   **c.** Fascia

18. a. Interstitial   **b.** Isthmus   **c.** Ampulla
d. Infundibulum with fimbriae

19. The lining of the uterine tubes is mucous membrane of <u>ciliated cubical epithelium</u> that is thrown into folds known as <u>plicae</u>. These folds <u>slow down</u> the ovum on its way to the uterus. There are <u>goblet cells</u> within the lining that produce a secretion containing <u>glycogen</u> to nourish the <u>oocyte</u>. The muscle coat consists of two layers, an inner <u>circular</u> layer and an outer <u>longitudinal</u> layer. Both layers are composed of <u>smooth muscle</u> which produce <u>peristaltic movement</u> of the tube.

20.

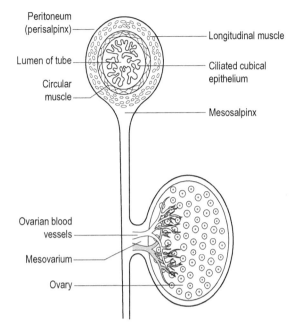

Figure 2.6

21.

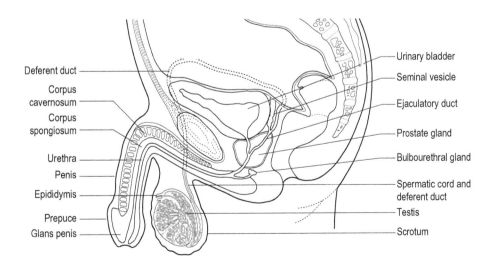

Figure 2.7

22. True – b, d, f, g, h, i

False – a, c, e

23. d.

24. a.

The female urinary tract

ANSWERS

1.

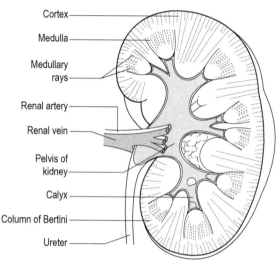

Figure 3.1

2. i. waste materials **ii.** toxins **iii.** water content
 iv. pH of blood **v.** the osmotic pressure of blood
 vi. hormones (renin and erythropoietin)

3. The glomerulus is fed by a branch of the renal
 artery, the **afferent** arteriole, and the blood is
 collected into the **efferent** arteriole. The pressure
 within the glomerulus is **raised** because the **afferent**
 arteriole has a wider bore than the **efferent**
 arteriole. This factor forces the filtrate **out of** the
 capillaries **into** the capsule. At this stage any
 substance with a **small** molecular size will be
 filtered out.

   The cup of the capsule is first attached to a tubule
 that has three distinct regions before joining the
 straight collecting duct receiving urine. The first
 region of the tubule is the twisting **proximal
 convoluted tubule**, the middle region is the straight
 loop of Henle, and the third region before joining
 the collecting duct is the twisting **distal convoluted
 tubule.**

4.

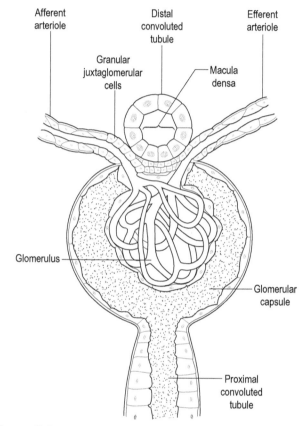

Figure 3.2

5.

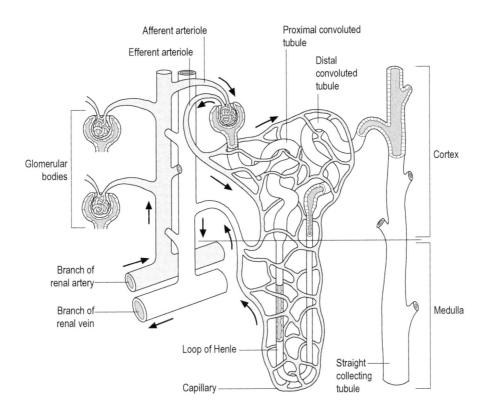

Figure 3.3

6. a. **7.** b. **8.** c. **9.** a. **10.** a. **11.** d. **12.** b.
13. d. **14.** b.

15.

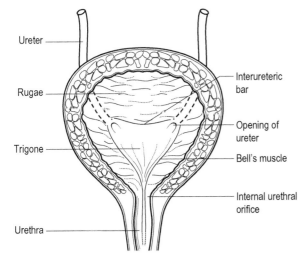

Figure 3.4

16. The ureters are composed of three layers: <u>a lining</u>, <u>a muscle layer</u> and an <u>outer coat</u>. At the upper end of the urinary tract, the ureter is continuous with the renal <u>hilum</u> of the kidney and runs to the <u>posterior</u> wall of the bladder. Each tube is about <u>3</u> mm in diameter and between <u>25</u> and <u>30</u> cm in length. The ureters transport urine to the bladder by <u>peristalsis</u>. The shape of the bladder is described as being <u>pyramidal</u> when empty and becomes more <u>globular</u> in shape as it becomes filled with urine. The base of the bladder is termed <u>trigone</u>. It is situated at the <u>back</u> of the bladder and rests against the <u>vagina</u>. The capacity of the bladder is around <u>600</u> ml.

17. a. Two pubovesical ligaments – Extend from: bladder neck anteriorly – To: <u>symphysis pubis</u>.

b. <u>Two lateral ligaments</u> – Extend from: <u>bladder</u> – To: the side walls of the pelvis.

c. <u>Urachas (single fibrous band)</u> – Extends from: apex of bladder – To: the <u>umbilicus</u>.

18. True: b, c, d, e, g, i, k, l, m, n, p, q

False: a, f, h, j, o

1. Phase One

In the **follicular** phase low levels of ovarian hormones stimulate the **hypothalamus** to produce **gonadotrophin releasing hormone (GnRH)**. This hormone causes the production of **follicle stimulating hormone (FSH)** and **luteinizing hormone** (LH) by the **anterior** pituitary gland. Under the influence of this hormone, the Graafian follicle secretes **oestrogen** and as a result there is a surge in **LH**. When hormone levels reach a certain peak, the secretion of **FSH** is inhibited. Eventually the largest and most dominant follicle secretes **inhibin**, which further suppresses **FSH**, and this follicle prevails and becomes competent to ovulate. The time from growth and maturity of the Graafian follicles to ovulation is normally around **one week**, day **5–14** of a 28-day cycle of events.

Phase Two

Ovulation is stimulated by a sudden **surge** in **LH** which matures the **oocyte**. This surge occurs around day **12–13** of a 28-day cycle and lasts for **48 hours**.

Phase Three

In the final **luteal** phase, the **corpus luteum** is formed by **proliferation** of the residual ruptured follicle. This is a **yellow** irregular structure producing **oestrogen** and **progesterone** for approximately **2** weeks. This develops the **endometrium** which awaits the fertilized oocyte. The **corpus luteum** continues its role until the **placenta** is developed adequately to take over. If fertilization does not occur then the **corpus luteum** degenerates and becomes the **corpus albicans.** There is a decrease in **oestrogen and progesterone** hormones and inhibitin levels. These low hormone levels stimulate the **hypothalamus** to produce **GnRH.** Rising levels of these hormones stimulate the **anterior** pituitary gland to produce **FSH** and the cycle begins again.

2.

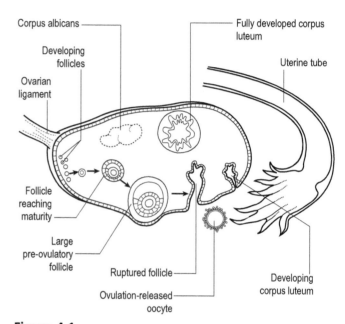

Corpus albicans
Developing follicles
Ovarian ligament
Follicle reaching maturity
Large pre-ovulatory follicle
Ruptured follicle
Ovulation-released oocyte
Fully developed corpus luteum
Uterine tube
Developing corpus luteum

Figure 4.1

3.

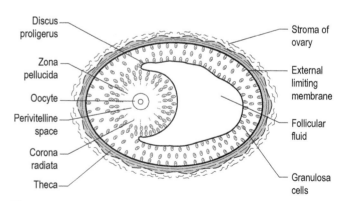

Discus proligerus
Zona pellucida
Oocyte
Perivitelline space
Corona radiata
Theca
Stroma of ovary
External limiting membrane
Follicular fluid
Granulosa cells

Figure 4.2

4.

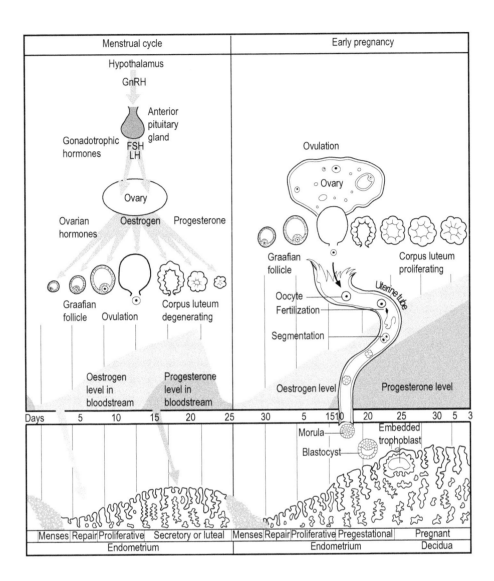

Figure 4.3

5. Menstrual phase: b, c, f, k, n, p

Proliferative phase: d, e, i, l, o, q, r

Secretory phase: a, g, h, j, m, s

6.

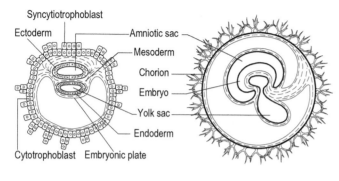

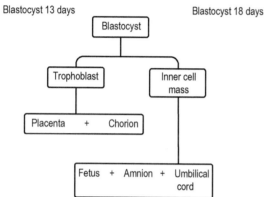

Figure 4.4

7. Once inside the uterine tubes the sperm undergo changes to the plasma membrane resulting in the removal of the glycoprotein coat. The **acrosomal** layer of the sperm becomes reactive with the release of the enzyme **hyaluronidase** and this is known as the **acrosome** reaction. This disperses the outermost layer of the oocyte called **corona radiata** allowing access to the **zona pellucida**. The first sperm that reaches the **zona pellucida** penetrates it with the aid of several enzymes. Upon penetration **cortical** reaction occurs which makes the **zona pellucida** impermeable to other sperm. The **plasma membranes** of the oocyte and sperm fuse. The oocyte at this stage completes its **second** meiotic division and becomes **mature**.

8. **a.** Haploid: On fusion of the sperm and oocyte, the pronucleus has 23 chromosomes and is referred to as haploid.

b. Diploid: The diploid cell contains the combination of the genetic material from both sperm and oocyte.

c. Zygote: The male and female gametes each contribute half of the complement of chromosomes to make a total of 46 (23 pairs) in the form of the new cell called the zygote. Two chromosomes are sex chromosomes.

9. During the journey along the uterine tube the zygote undergoes <u>mitotic</u> cellular replication and division referred to as <u>cleavage</u> resulting in smaller cells known as <u>blastomeres</u>. The zygote divides into two cells at day 1, four at day 2, eight by 2.5 days and sixteen by 3 days, now known as the <u>morula</u>. The cells bind together in a process known as <u>compaction</u>. Next <u>cavitation</u> occurs whereby the outermost cells secrete fluid into the <u>morula</u> and a fluid filled cavity or <u>blastocele</u> appears in the <u>morula</u>. This results in the formation of the <u>blastocyst</u> that enters the <u>uterus</u> around day 3–5. The <u>blastocyst</u> possesses an <u>inner cell mass</u> or <u>embryoblast</u> and an <u>outer cell mass</u> or <u>trophoblast</u>. Implantation of the <u>trophoblast</u> layer occurs into the endometrium, which at this point becomes known as the <u>decidua</u>. The <u>outer cell mass</u> or <u>trophoblast</u> becomes the <u>placenta</u> and chorion while the <u>inner cell mass</u> or <u>embryoblast</u> becomes the <u>embryo</u>, <u>amnion</u> and umbilical cord.

10. **a.** Ectoderm – This is the start of the tissue that covers most of the body surfaces – the epidermis layer of the skin, hair, nails. It also forms the nervous system.

b. Mesoderm – This forms the muscle, skeleton, connective tissue, blood vessels and blood, lymph cells, the urogenital glands and dermis of the skin.

c. Endoderm – This forms the epithelia lining of the respiratory, digestive, urinary systems and the glandular cells of organs such as liver and pancreas.

11. True: a, b, c, d, e, f, i, k, m, n, o

    False: g, h, j, l

12. b.   13. c.   14. d.   15. c.

1.

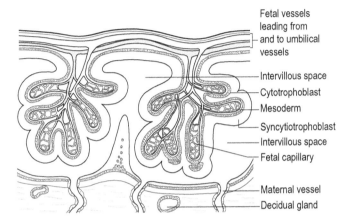

Fetal vessels leading from and to umbilical vessels

Intervillous space

Cytotrophoblast

Mesoderm

Syncytiotrophoblast

Intervillous space

Fetal capillary

Maternal vessel

Decidual gland

Figure 5.1

2.

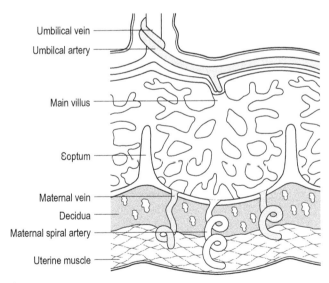

Umbilical vein

Umbilcal artery

Main villus

Septum

Maternal vein

Decidua

Maternal spiral artery

Uterine muscle

Figure 5.2

3. a. By 10 days, the blastocyst is completely buried in the decidua. The trophoblasts have a potent invasive capacity. The decidua secretes cytokines and protease inhibitors that moderate this invasion.

↓

b. Chorionic villi form from the proliferation of projections from the trophoblastic layer from about 3 weeks after fertilization. This becomes more profuse in the decidua basilis where there is a rich blood supply. This is known as the chorion frondosum which develops into the placenta.

↓

c. The portion of deciduas surrounding the blastocyst where it projects into the uterine cavity is known as the decidua capsularis. The vili under this area degenerates forming chorion laeve from where the chorionic membrane originates. The remaining decidua is known as the decidua parietalis.

↓

d. As the uterus is filled with the enlarging fetus the decidua capsularis thins and disappears and the chorion meets the decidua parietalis on the opposite wall of the uterus.

↓

e. The villi penetrate the decidua and erode the walls of maternal blood vessels opening them up to form a lake of maternal blood in which they float. The opened blood vessels are known as sinuses and the area surrounding the villi are called blood spaces.

4. Respiration, nutrition, excretion, storage, protection, and endocrine. (The placenta also provides placental circulation.)

5. Maternal blood is discharged into the intervillous space by **80–100** spiral arteries. Blood flows **slowly** around the villi, eventually returning to the endometrial **veins** and the maternal circulation. There are about **150 mL** of maternal blood in the intervillous spaces, which is exchanged **3 or 4** times per minute.

Fetal blood, **low** in oxygen, is pumped by the fetal heart towards the placenta along the umbilical **arteries** and transported along their branches to the capillaries of the chorionic villi where exchange of nutrients takes place between mother and fetus. Having yielded up **carbon dioxide** and waste products and absorbed **oxygen** and nutrients the blood is returned to the fetus via the umbilical **vein**.

6. True: b, c, d, g, h, i, j

False: a, e, f

7. Anchoring villi and nutritive villi.

8. Treponema of syphilis **or** tubercle bacillus.

9. Rubella **and** human cytomegalovirus.

10. Human chorionic gonadotrophin (HCG), oestrogens, progesterone, human placental lactogen (hPL).

11. a–iii b–iv c–v d–ii e–vi f–i

12. i. Chorion: a, e, h, i, j

ii. Amnion: c, b, d, f, g, k, l

13. a. During pregnancy: Equalizes pressure, allows normal growth and free movement of the fetus; protects the fetus from injury; maintains a constant temperature; prevents fetal heat loss and has a small nutritional function.

b. In labour: Protects the placenta and umbilical cord from pressure during uterine contractions, aids effacement of the cervix and aids dilatation of the uterine os.

14. a. 20 cm **b.** 2.5 cm **c.** one-sixth

15. Maternal surface: c, e, g, i, j

Fetal surface: a, b, d, f, h

16. a. i. Three

ii. One umbilical vein and two umbilical arteries

b. Wharton's jelly

c. i. 1–2 cm

ii. 40–50 cm

d. Occlusion of blood vessels through knotting of cord or being wrapped around the neck or body of fetus.

17. a.

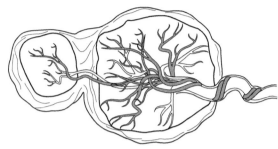

Figure 5.3 Succenturiate lobe of placenta.

It is a succenturiate lobe of placenta. A small extra lobe is present but separate from the main placenta and joined to it by blood vessels that run through the membranes that reach it.

Associated risk factors: A small lobe may be retained in utero following delivery of the placenta. This may lead to infection and haemorrhage.

b.

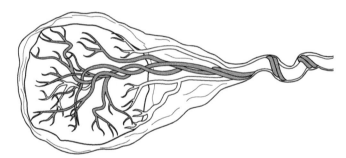

Figure 5.4 Velamentous placenta.

A velamentous insertion of the cord occurs when the cord is inserted into the membranes some distance from the edge of the placenta. The umbilical vessels run through the membranes from the cord to placenta.

Associated risk factors: In placentae that are low lying then the vessels may pass across the uterine os (vasa praevia). There is a risk to the fetus when membranes rupture, as vessels may be torn, leading to rapid exsanguination of the fetus.

18. b. **19.** c. **20.** c. **21.** d. **22.** b. **23.** b.

1. 0–4 weeks: b, c   4–8 weeks: m   8–12 weeks: d, g, h, l
12–16 weeks: a, f, k   16–20 weeks: e, i, j

2. 20–24 weeks: c, e   24–28 weeks: d, f   28–32 weeks:
a, g   32–36 wks: b, h, j, k, l   36 weeks–birth: i

3.

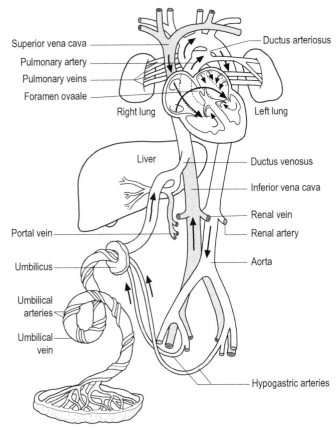

Figure 6.1

4. **a.** umbilical vein, inferior vena cava

   b. pulmonary artery

   c. right and left atria

   d. internal iliac arteries, umbilical arteries

5. **a.** Oxygenated blood from the placenta travels **to** the fetus in the **umbilical vein**. The **umbilical vein** divides into two branches: one that supplies the **portal vein** in the liver, the other the **ductus venosus** joining the **inferior** vena cava.

b. Most of the oxygenated blood that enters the **right** atrium passes across the foramen ovale to the **left** atrium and from here into the **left** ventricle, and then to the **aorta**. The head and **upper** extremities receive about half of the blood supply via the coronary and carotid arteries, and subclavian arteries respectively. The remainder of blood travels in the **descending aorta**, mixing with **deoxygenated** blood from the **right** ventricle.

c. Deoxygenated blood collected from the upper parts of the body returns to the **right** atrium in the **superior** vena cava.

Blood that has entered the **right** atrium from the inferior and superior vena cava passes into the **right** ventricle. A small amount of blood travels to the lungs in the **pulmonary artery** for their development.

d. Most blood passes through the ductus **arteriosus** into the **descending** aorta. **Deoxygenated blood** travels back to the placenta via the **internal** iliac arteries leading into the hypogastric **arteries** which lead into the umbilical **arteries.**

6. **a.** ligamentum teres

   b. ligamentum venosum

   c. ligamentum arteriosum

   d. obliterated hypogastric arteries, superior vesical arteries

   e. fossa ovalis

7. b.   **8.** d.   **9.** c.   **10.** a.   **11.** d.   **12.** c.

13. a. Protect the vital centres in the medulla

b. 14, non-compressible

c. Orbital ridges, nape of the neck

d. It relates to the process involved in laying down of the bones of the vault from the ossification centres

e. Key ossification centres: i. Occipital protuberance, ii. Parietal eminence, iii. Frontal eminence

f. A suture is a cranial joint formed where two bones meet

g. A fontanelle is formed where two or more sutures meet

14. a. Occipital bone, Lies at the back of the head, Occipital protuberance

b. Two parietal bones, Lie on either side of the skull, Parietal eminences

c. Two frontal bones, Form the forehead and sinciput, Frontal eminence

15. a. Lambdoidal suture, Separates the occipital bone from the two parietal bones

b. Sagittal suture, Lies between the two parietal bones, passing from one temple to the other

c. Coronal suture, Separates the frontal bones from the parietal bones, passing from one temple to the other

d. Frontal suture, Runs between the two halves of the frontal bone

16. a. Posterior fontanelle (or lambda); Small, triangular, shaped like the Greek letter Lambda λ; Situated at the junction of the lambdoidal and sagittal sutures; 6 weeks

b. Anterior fontanelle (or bregma); Broad, kite-shaped, 3–4 cm long and 1.5–2 cm wide; Found at the junction of the sagittal, coronal and frontal sutures; 18 months

17.

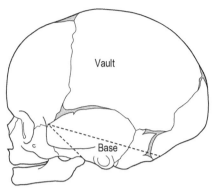

Figure 6.2

18.

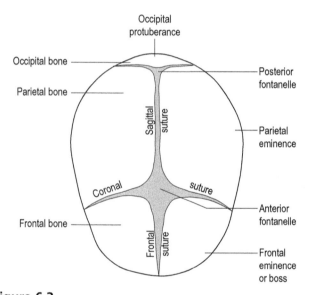

Figure 6.3

19. a. Occiput region, Lies between the <u>foramen magnum</u> and <u>posterior fontanelle</u>. The part below the <u>occipital protuberance</u> (landmark) is known as the sub-occipital region.

b. Vertex region, This region is bounded by the posterior fontanelle, the two <u>parietal eminences</u> and anterior fontanelle.

c. Forehead/sinciput region, Extends from the anterior fontanelle and the <u>coronal suture</u> to the <u>orbital ridges</u>.

d. Face, Extends from orbital ridges and the <u>root</u> of the <u>nose</u> to the junction of the chin or <u>mentum</u> (landmark) and the neck. The point between the eyebrows is known as the <u>glabella</u> (landmark).

20.

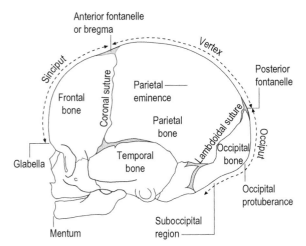

Figure 6.4

23.

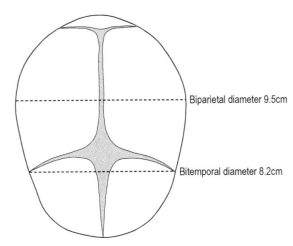

Biparietal diameter 9.5cm

Bitemporal diameter 8.2cm

Figure 6.5

21. **a.** Sub-occipitobregmatic (SOB), From below the occipital protuberance to the centre of the anterior fontanelle (bregma), 9.5 cm.

b. Sub-occipitofrontal (SOF), From below the occipital protuberance to the centre of the frontal suture, 10 cm

c. Occipitofrontal (OF), From the occipital protuberance to the glabella, 11.5 cm.

d. Mentovertical (MV), From the point of the chin to the highest point on the vertex (slightly nearer to the posterior than the anterior fontanelle), 13.5 cm.

e. Sub-mentovertical (SMV), From the point where the chin joins the neck to the highest point on the vertex, 11.5 cm.

f. Sub-mentobregmatic (SMB), From the point where the chin joins the neck to the centre of the bregma, 9.5 cm.

22. **a.** The bisacromial diameter (12 cm): This is the distance between the acromion processes on the shoulder blades.

b. Bitrochanteric diameter (10 cm): This is measured between the greater trochanters of the femurs.

24. **a.** Vertex presentation:

When the head is well flexed the sub-occipitobregmatic diameter (9.5 cm) and the biparietal diameter (9.5 cm) present. The sub-occipitofrontal diameter (10 cm) distends the vaginal orifice.

When the head is deflexed, the presenting diameters are the occipitofrontal (11.5 cm) and the biparietal (9.5 cm). This often arises when the occiput is in a posterior position. If this remains then the occipitofrontal diameter (11.5 cm) distends the vaginal orifice.

b. Face presentation:

When the head is completely extended the presenting diameters are the sub-mentobregmatic (9.5 cm) and the bitemporal (8.2 cm). The sub-mentovertical diameter (11.5 cm) will distend the vaginal orifice.

c. Brow presentation:

This occurs when the head is partially extended and the mentovertical diameter (13.5 cm) and bitemporal diameter (8.2 cm) present. Vaginal birth is unlikely.

25. a. Moulding is used to describe the change in shape of the fetal head that takes place during its passage through the birth canal.

b. The bones of the vault allow a slight degree of bending. The skull bones are soft and able to override at the sutures.

26.

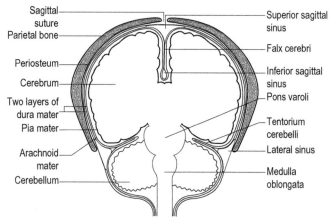

Figure 6.6

27.

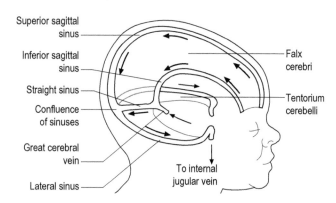

Figure 6.7

28. a.   **29.** d.   **30.** b.

Change and adaptation in pregnancy

ANSWERS

1. **a.** 3–4 weeks+ **c.** 4–14 weeks **d.** 6–12 weeks
   e. 16–20 weeks+ **f.** Human chorionic
   gonadotrophin hormone (hCG) **g.** 9–10 days
   h. 14 days **i.** 8 weeks+ **j.** 5.5 weeks
   k. 11–12 weeks **l.** 20 weeks+ **m.** 22 weeks+
   n. 24 weeks+

2. True: a, c, e, g

   False: b, d, f, h

3. **a.** 1100 g

   b. 30 × 22.5 × 20 cm

4. **a.** 38 **b.** 36 **c.** 20 **d.** increased vascularity and
   oedema **e.** internal os, lowest **f.** endocervical
   mucosal, tenacious mucus.

5. Cervical ripening involves **inflammatory** cells but is
   likely dependent upon **endogenously** produced
   prostaglandins. Rearrangement and degradation of
   collagen fibres creates an **increase** in the space
   between them, **shortens** them and **increases** acidic
   solubility along with **reduced** capacity to **retain**
   water. The cervix changes to a **soft distensible**
   structure with **reduced** resistance to effacement and
   dilatation.

6. **a.** The uterine souffle refers to the <u>soft blowing</u>
   sound made by the blood passing through the
   <u>dilated uterine vessels</u> and heard distinctly at the
   lower portion of the uterus. The souffle is
   synchronous with the <u>maternal pulse</u>.

b. The placental souffle refers to the <u>muffled
'ocean-like'</u> sound of blood coursing through the
<u>placenta</u>. This is synchronous with the <u>fetal heart</u>.

c. 'Chadwick's sign refers to violet or dark purplish
<u>discolouration</u> and <u>congestion</u> of the vulva and
<u>vaginal</u> mucous membranes. This is due to
<u>increased</u> vascularity and is first detected between
the <u>4</u>th and <u>8</u>th week of pregnancy.

d. <u>Osiander's</u> sign refers to the stronger and harder
vaginal pulsations in the fornices caused by the
increased blood supply and enlarged uterine artery.

e. Leuccorrhoea refers to the thick, white <u>vaginal</u>
discharge and is due to the high levels of <u>oestrogen</u>.

7. c. **8.** b. **9.** c. **10.** c. **11.** d. **12.** a.

13. **a. Increases** in size, shifted **upwards** and to the
    left.

    b. Dramatic systemic and pulmonary vasodilation
    to **increase** blood flow.

    c. Increased permeability.

    d. Vasodilation and impeded **venous** return in
    lower extremities.

    e. Haemodilution, increased capacity for clot
    formation.

14.

Parameter	Adaptation (↑,↔,↓, etc.)	Magnitude of change (%, etc.)	Non-pregnant (average value)	Timing of peak: average peak value
Plasma volume	↑	50%	2600 mL	**32 weeks: 3850 mL**
Red cell mass	↑	N/A	1400 mL	30 weeks: **1550 mL**
Total blood volume	↑	30–45%	**4000 mL**	32 weeks: 4600 mL
Cardiac output	↑	35–50%	4.9 L/min	**28 weeks; 7 L/min**
Stroke volume	↑	N/A	N/A	**20 weeks**
Heart rate	↑	10–15 bpm	75 bpm	**Trimester 1: 90 bpm**
Systemic vascular resistance	↓	21%	N/A	Trimester 2
Pulmonary vascular resistance	↓	35%	N/A	**34 weeks**
Diastolic blood pressure	↓ returning to normal by term	10–15 mmHg	N/A	24 weeks
Systemic blood pressure	Minimal, no ↓	5–10 mmHg	N/A	24 weeks
Serum colloid osmotic pressure	↓	10–15%	N/A	14 weeks

15. True: a, b, d

False: c

16. a. Supine hypotensive syndrome occurs when the enlarging uterus compresses both the inferior vena cava and the lower aorta when the woman lies supine.

b. Hypotension, bradycardia, dizziness, light-headedness, nausea, and possible syncope.

c. Compression of the aorta may lead to reduced uteroplacental and renal blood flow and fetal compromise, loss of consciousness due to a decrease in blood pressure and cerebral blood flow.

17. Non-pregnant:

Haemoglobin (g/dL): 11.5–16.5

Pregnant (typical range):

Urea (mmol/L): usually ≤ 4.5   Albumin (g/L): 25–35   Potassium (mmol/L): unchanged

Clotting time (min): 8   Fibrinogen (g/L): By term 2.9–6.2

Haemoglobin (g/dL): 10.0–12.0   Alanine transaminase (ALT) (U/L): 6–40 U/L; no change

Platelets (x10⁹L): slight decrease in normal pregnancy; Lower limits of 'normal' = 120

18. a. 'Apparent anaemia' – despite the increased number of red blood cells, the marked increase in plasma volume causes dilution of many circulating factors. As a result red cell count, haematocrit and haemoglobin concentrations all decrease.

b. Blood viscosity is reduced, leading to reduced resistance to blood flow. This improves placental perfusion and reduced maternal cardiac effort.

19. True: a, e

False: b, c, d

20. a. The increased tendency to clot is caused by increases in clotting factors and fibrinogen.

b. From 12 weeks' gestation there is a 50% increase in the synthesis of plasma fibrinogen (factor I).

c. Coagulation factors VII, VIII and X increase during pregnancy.

21. Increase: a, b, c, d, f, h

Decrease: e, g

22. True: b, c, d, e, i

False: a, f, g, h.

23. Dilatation of the ureters, which is rarely present **below** the pelvic brim, is possibly due to compression by the enlarging uterus and **ovarian plexus**. The early onset of ureteral dilatation suggests that smooth muscle relaxation, caused by **progesterone**, possibly plays an additional role. The dilatation is more marked on the **right** side, due to the cushioning effect of the **sigmoid** colon on the **left** and due to the uterine tendency to **dextrorotation**.

24. Pica is the persistent craving and compulsive consumption of unusual substances. Examples of the substances consumed include clay, soap, coal or starch. Pica can cause a number of medical problems, such as nutritional deficiencies, constipation, electrolyte imbalance, gastrointestinal and metabolic disturbances, lead poisoning, dental complications and weight gain. There are two main viewpoints about the origins of pica practices and these include:

1. It has cultural roots.
2. It is a behavioural response to stress, a habit or disorder, or a manifestation of an oral fixation.

25. In late pregnancy, although basal insulin levels are **elevated,** maternal blood glucose levels are similar to non-pregnant levels and do not **reduce** as rapidly as usual even with **higher** circulating levels of insulin. This diabetogenic state protects the fetus even if the mother is fasting by keeping glucose in the blood and thus available for placental transfer. After a meal, however, the pregnant woman's levels of gluscose and insulin are **higher** than those of non-pregnant women and **glycogen** is suppressed resulting in **hyper-**insulinaemia, **hyper-**glycaemia and insulin resistance.

26. Maternal weight (kg):

Uterus (0.9 kg)   Breasts (0.4 kg)   Fat (4.0 kg)
     Blood (1.2 kg)   Extracellular fluid (1.2 kg)

Total for maternal (7.7 kg)

Fetal weight (kg):

Fetus (3.3 kg)   Placenta (0.7 kg)   Amniotic fluid (0.8 kg)

Total for fetal weight (4.8 kg)

Grand total 12.5 kg   Percentage of total weight: maternal 64%, fetal 36%

27. Relaxation of the pelvic joints is predominantly due to hormonal influences. The hormone oestrogen modifies the connective tissue making it more pliable. This causes the joint capsules to relax, making the pelvic joints mobile. The hormone progesterone has the effect of relaxing or weakening the pelvic ligaments. The hormone relaxin plays a major role in the changes, remodelling collagen fibres and softening pelvic joints and ligaments in preparation for birth.

28. a. 3 kg in the first trimester followed by 0.4 kg per week for the remainder of the pregnancy.

b. Sacroiliac and sacrococcygeal joints.

c. Pigmentation of the face caused by melanin deposition into epidermal and dermal macrophages.

d. The 'mask of pregnancy'.

e. Hyperpigmentation, some degree of skin darkening, linea nigra, striae gravidarum (stretch marks), pruritus, peripheral vasodilation, acceleration of sweat gland activity, angiomas or vascular spiders (on face, neck, arms and chest), palmar erythema.

29. 3–4 weeks: Prickling, tingling sensation, particularly around the nipple. Due to increased blood supply.

6–8 weeks: Increase in size, painful, tense and nodular, delicate, bluish surface, veins become visible just beneath the skin. Due to hypertrophy of the alveoli.

8–12 weeks: Montgomery tubercles become more prominent on the areola. The pigmented area around the nipple (primary areola) darkens and may become more erectile. Hypertrophic sebaceous glands secrete sebum, which keeps the nipple soft. Increased melanin activity.

16 weeks: Colostrum can be expressed. The secondary areola develops with further extension of the pigmented area which is often mottled in appearance.

Late pregnancy: Colostrum may leak from the breast. The nipple becomes more prominent and mobile. Progesterone causes the nipple to become more prominent and mobile.

30. a. Epulis is a specific angiogranuloma, which can be caused by advanced gingivitis.

b. Leptin is a peptide hormone, secreted by both placental and adipose tissue and plays a key role in the regulation of body fat and energy expenditure.

c. In the posterior maternal and fetal pituitary glands, myometrium, decidua, placenta and fetal membranes.

d. Stimulates contractions in the myometrium, causes contractions in the myoepithelial cells of the breast to eject milk following birth.

e. In the anterior pituitary (for the majority), breasts, decidua and is found in high concentrations in amniotic fluid.

f. It promotes mammary development and stimulates lactation.

31. d.   **32.** a.   **33.** a.   **34.** d.   **35.** d.   **36.** d.   **37.** a.
38. b.   **39.** a.   **40.** a.

1. **a.** Naegele's rule is the estimated date of delivery (EDD) calculated by adding 9 calendar months and 7 days to the date of the first day of the woman's menstrual period.

   b. Conception occurred 14 days after the first day of the last period; this is true only if the woman has a regular 28 day cycle. The woman has recorded regularity and length of time between periods. The last period of bleeding was true menstruation (implantation of the ovum may cause bleeding). Breakthrough bleeding and anovulation can be affected by the contraceptive pill thus impacting on the accuracy of a LMP.

2. **a.** <18.5 kg/m^2 **b.** 18.5 – 24.9 kg/m^2 **c.** 25.0 – 29.9 kg/m^2 **d.** 30–39.9 kg/m^2 **e.** ≥40 kg/m^2

3. **a.** Ketonuria – ketones are due to the breakdown of fat. Ketonuria may be due to a variety of reasons including vomiting, hyperemesis, starvation or excessive exercise.

   b. Proteinuria – this may be caused by contamination by vaginal leucorrhoea, or hypertensive disorders of pregnancy.

4. **a.** Routine blood tests: ABO blood group and rhesus factor, full blood count, venereal disease research laboratory (VDRL), rubella immune status, HIV antibodies (it is now recommended that this test is routinely offered to women).

   b. Possible other blood tests: HIV antibodies (it is now recommended that this test is routinely offered to women), hepatitis B, screening tests for other blood disorders, e.g. sickle cell anaemia or thalassaemias.

5. **a.** Engagement has occurred when the widest presenting transverse diameter has passed through the brim of the pelvis.

   b. i. biparietal 9.5 cm

   ii. bitrochanteric 10 cm

   c. Normally from the 36th week onwards

   d. Malposition, cephalopelvic disproportion, occipitoposterior position, full bladder, wrongly calculated gestational age, polyhydramnios, placenta praevia (or other lesion occupying the space), multiple pregnancy, pelvic abnormalities, fetal abnormalities.

6. **a.** The part of the fetus that lies at the pelvic brim or in the lower pole of the uterus.

   b. Is the relationship between the long axis of the fetus and the long axis of the uterus.

   c. Is the relationship of the fetal head and limbs to its trunk.

   d. i. To 'give name to'.

   ii. Is the name of the part of the presentation which is used when referring to fetal position.

   e. The relationship between the denominator of the presentation and six points of the pelvic brim.

7. **a.** Longitudinal lie, oblique lie, transverse lie.

   b. The preferred attitude is <u>one of flexion</u>. The fetus <u>is curled up with chin on chest, arms and legs flexed, forming a snug, compact mass which utilizes the space in the uterine cavity most effectively</u>.

   c. i. mentum

   ii. sacrum

   iii. occiput

8. a–ii b–vi c–iii d–i e–v f–viii g–vii h–iv

9.

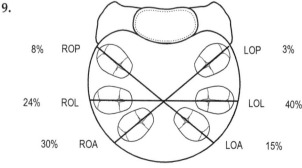

8%	ROP		LOP	3%
24%	ROL		LOL	40%
30%	ROA		LOA	15%

Figure 8.1

10. a. Increasing uterine size in comparison with the gestational age of the fetus.

b. Fetal movements that follow a regular pattern from the time when they are first felt.

c. Fetal heart rate that is regular and variable with a rate between 110 and 160 bpm.

11. True: a, b, e, f, g, h, j, k, l

False: c, d, i, m

12. Neural tube defects, multiple pregnancies, incorrect gestation, threatened miscarriage

13. Spine, head shape and internal structures, abdominal shape and content (at level of stomach), abdominal shape and content (at level of kidneys and umbilicus), renal pelvis (<5 mm), longitudinal axis, abdominal-thoracic appearance (diaphragm and bladder), thorax – at level of four chamber cardiac view, arms – three bones and hand, legs – three bones and foot, face and lips and cardiac output tracts.

14. Hypothermia, hypoglycaemia and premature birth.

15. It is the thickness of the subcutaneous collection of fluid at the back of the neck. NT at 10–14 weeks' gestation provides additional information about the fetus.

16. Fluorescent in situ hybridization (FISH), quanatitative fluorescence-polymerase chain reaction (QF-PCR).

17. Fetal imaging technique, fetal cells in the maternal circulation, fetal therapy, e.g. therapeutic amniocentesis.

18. d.   **19.** b.   **20.** e.   **21.** c.   **22.** c.   **23.** a.

1. **a.** a small amount of bleeding occurring as the blastocyst implants into the endometrium 5–7 days after fertilization.

   b. termination of pregnancy prior to 24 weeks' gestation or a fetal weight of < 500 g.

   c. three or more successive pregnancy losses prior to viability.

   d. any pregnancy occurring outside the uterine cavity.

2. Genetic abnormalities, endocrine factors, maternal illness and infection, abnormalities of the uterus, cervical incompetence, autoimmune factors and thrombophilic defects and alloimmune factors.

3. Threatened miscarriage, inevitable/incomplete miscarriage, complete miscarriage, missed or silent miscarriage, miscarriage with infection.

4. **a.** Uterine and adnexal tenderness, purulent vaginal loss and pyrexia.

   b. Endotoxic shock, fatal hypotension, renal failure, disseminated intravascular coagulopathy, and multiple petechial haemorrhages.

   c. *Escherichia coli, Streptococcus faecalis, Staphylococcus albus* and *aureus, Klebsiella, Clostridium welchii* and *C. perfringens.*

5.

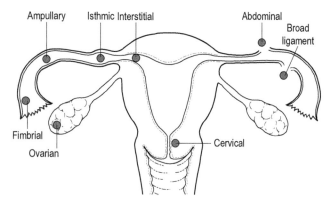

Figure 9.1

6. **a.** Amenorrhoea, lower abdominal pain of sudden onset starting locally and becoming generalized as blood loss extends into the peritoneal cavity, sub-diaphragmatic irritation by blood produces referred shoulder tip pain and discomfort on breathing. There may be episodes of syncope.

   b. Hypotension, tachycardia and signs of peritonism including abdominal distension, guarding, rebound tenderness. On pelvic examination the cervix is closed and acutely tender when moved due to irritation of the pelvic peritoneum caused by bleeding.

7. Molar pregnancy most commonly presents with <u>bleeding</u> in <u>the first half of</u> pregnancy. It is usually diagnosed initially as a <u>threatened</u> miscarriage. The uterus is <u>larger</u> than dates in about half of the cases. On ultrasound examination a '<u>snowstorm</u>' appearance usually suggests molar disease. Associated conditions include: unexplained <u>anaemia</u>, severe <u>hyperemesis</u>, <u>pre-eclampsia</u>, and <u>ovarian cysts</u>.

8. **a.** persistent pregnancy-related vomiting associated with weight loss of >5% of body mass and ketosis.

   b. tachycardia, hypotension and loss of skin turgor.

   c. encephalopathy, renal and hepatic failure.

9. Incarceration of retroversion of the uterus, ovarian cysts, fibroids.

10. True: a, b, e, f

    False: c, d

11. b.   **12.** b.   **13.** c.

14. **a.** Pelvic girdle pain (PGP) is also known as <u>symphysis pubis dysfunction</u> (<u>SPD</u>). It is characterized by <u>abnormal relaxation of the ligaments supporting the pubic joint</u>. This is brought about by several factors including <u>high</u>

levels of pregnancy hormones *(particularly relaxin, biochemical and genetic factors)*. It affects 1 in <u>300</u> women.

b. Antepartum haemorrhage refers to <u>bleeding from the genital tract in late pregnancy after the 24th weeks of gestation and before labour.</u>

c. The condition known as placenta praevia refers to <u>the placenta being partially or wholly implanted in the lower uterine segment on either the anterior or posterior wall.</u>

d. Placenta abruption is defined as <u>premature separation of a normally situated placenta occurring after the 22nd week of pregnancy.</u>

e. Blood loss from a placental abruption may be defined as being <u>revealed</u>, <u>concealed</u> or <u>mixed</u> haemorrhages.

15. This occurs in placental abruption when blood is retained behind the placenta. It may be forced into the myometrium and it infiltrates between the muscle fibres. This extravasation can cause marked damage. There is no vaginal bleeding, the mother will have all the signs and symptoms of hypovolaemic shock (reduced cardiac output, drop in BP, increased heart rate, pale, cool and moist skin, dilatation of the pupils of the eyes) caused by the concealed bleeding into the uterine muscles. The concealed haemorrhage causes uterine enlargement and extreme pain.

16. Type 1: f, j, l   Type 2: b, d, h, i, m   Type 3: a, g, k
    Type 4: c, e, n

17. True: a, b, c, f

    False: d, e

18. Normal blood clotting occurs in three main stages: 1. When tissues are damaged and <u>platelets</u> break down, <u>thromboplastin</u> is released; 2. In the presence of calcium ions, <u>thromboplastin</u> leads to the conversion of <u>prothrombin</u> into <u>thrombin</u>; 3. Thrombin is a proteolytic (protein-splitting) enzyme that converts <u>fibrinogen</u> into fibrin.

    <u>Fibrin</u> forms a network of long-sticky strands that entrap blood cells to form a <u>clot.</u> The coagulated material contracts and exudes a serum which is <u>plasma</u> depleted of <u>clotting factors</u>. The <u>coagulation mechanism</u> is normally held at bay by the presence of <u>heparin</u> which is produced in the liver.

    <u>Fibrinolysis</u> is the breakdown of fibrin and occurs in response to the presence of clotted blood. Coagulation will continue unless <u>fibrinolysis</u> takes place.

19. Placental abruption, intrauterine fetal death, amniotic fluid embolism, intrauterine infection, pre-eclampsia and eclampsia.

20. e.   21. c.   22. a.

23. True: a, c, e, f, h

    False: b, d, g

24. **a.** 1 L   **b.** 800 mL at term   **c.** 30 **d.** 20, monozygote twins or severe fetal abnormality   **e.** 300–500 mL

25. c.   26. a.   27. a.   28. b.

1. **a.** The term 'diabetes mellitus' describes a **metabolic** disorder that affects the normal **metabolism** of **carbohydrates**. It is characterized by **hyperglycaemia** and **glycosuria** resulting from defects in **insulin** secretion or action, or both. The classic signs and symptoms are **excessive thirst, excessive urinary excretion** and **unexplained weight loss**. The long term effects include **peripheral arterial disease, kidney disease, loss of vision, coronary heart disease, nerve damage**.

   b. Type 1 diabetes – This occurs when **beta** cells in the **islets of Langerhans** located in the **pancreas** are destroyed, stopping the production of **insulin**. Type 2 diabetes – This results from a **defect** in the action of **insulin**. The risk of developing this type of diabetes increases with, age, **obesity,** and **lack of physical activity**. Gestational diabetes (GDM) – This is defined as **carbohydrate intolerance** resulting in **hyperglycaemia** of variable severity. Onset or first recognition occurs during **pregnancy**.

   c. i. <6.1 mmol/L. ii. <2.2 mmol/L. iii. >25.0 mmol/L. iv. >7.8 mmol/L. v. >6.1 mmol/L and <7.0 mmol/L

2. Signs: pallor of mucus membrane. Symptoms: headache, shortness of breath on exertion, tachycardia, palpitations, fatigue, dizziness and fainting.

3. True: a, b, c, g, h, i, j, k, l

   False: d, e, f

4. **a.** 5. **d.** 6. **c.** 7. **a.** 8. **a.** 9. **c.**

10. **a.** This is known as hypertension <u>before</u> pregnancy or a <u>diastolic</u> blood pressure of <u>90</u> mmHg pre-pregnancy or before <u>20</u> weeks' gestation.

   b. This is the development of hypertension at or after <u>20</u> weeks' gestation when the woman's <u>diastolic</u> blood pressure was <<u>90</u> mmHg before <u>20</u> weeks' gestation. There are no other signs of pre-eclampsia.

   c. This is the presence of <u>proteinuria</u> defined as <u>1</u>+ (300 mg/L or more) on dipstick testing, a protein-creatinine ratio of ≥<u>30</u> mg/mmol on a random sample, or a urine <u>proteinuria</u> excretion of ≥300 mg/<u>24</u> hours.

   d. This is diagnosed on the basis of new hypertension with significant <u>proteinuria</u> at or after <u>20</u> weeks' gestation. Pre-eclampsia is a <u>multi-system</u> disorder, which can affect the <u>placenta</u>, <u>kidney</u>, brain, and other organs. In the absence of <u>proteinuria</u>, pre-eclampsia is suspected when <u>hypertension</u> is accompanied by symptoms including <u>headache</u>, blurred vision, <u>upper abdominal</u> pain, or altered biochemistry: specifically <u>raised</u> urates, <u>low</u> platelet counts and abnormal <u>liver</u> enzyme levels. These signs and symptoms together with blood pressure ><u>160</u> mmHg systolic or ><u>110</u> mmHg diastolic and proteinuria of <u>2</u>+ or <u>3</u>+ on a dipstick, demonstrate the more severe form of pre-eclampsia.

   e. This is defined as the new onset of <u>seizures</u> during pregnancy or postpartum, unrelated to other <u>cerebral</u> pathological conditions, in a woman with pre-eclampsia.

   f. The development of pre-eclampsia in women with pre-existing <u>hypertension</u> and/or pre-existing <u>proteinuria</u>.

11. **a.** increased **b.** increased
    c. thrombocytopenia **d.** prolonged **e.** raised

12. Haematocrit: <u>33–39</u>%, Platelets: <u>150–400</u> × 10⁹/L, Fibrinogen: <u>3.63–4.23</u> g/L

13. True: a, c, d, e, f, i, j

    False: b, g, h

14. **a.** H: Haemolysis, EL: Elevated Liver enzymes, LP: Low Platelet count

    b. HELLP syndrome typically manifests itself between <u>32</u> and <u>34</u> weeks' gestation. Of all cases, <u>30</u>% will occur postpartum with the onset typically being within <u>48</u> hours following birth. Women with HELLP syndrome will often complain of several symptoms including <u>malaise</u>, <u>nausea</u> and <u>vomiting</u>, <u>upper</u> abdominal pain with <u>tenderness</u>. Some women will experience non-specific viral-like symptoms. Investigations include <u>full blood count</u>, platelet count and liver function tests. These should be carried out irrespective of <u>maternal blood pressure</u> readings. Serious maternal complications include i. <u>abruptio</u> placentae, ii. disseminated <u>intravascular coagulation</u>, iii. eclampsia, iv. acute <u>renal failure</u> and v. sub-capsular haematoma of the <u>liver</u>.

15. Blood pressure –There is a **sharp rise** in BP; Headache – this is described as being **severe** and **persistent**. It is usually located in the **frontal** region. This is due to **cerebral vasospasm**. Level of consciousness – The woman is <u>drowsy</u> and **confused**. This is due to **cerebral vasospasm**. Visual – There are visual **disturbances** such as **blurring of vision** and **blindness**. This is due to **cerebral vasospasm**. Urinary output – output is **diminished**. There may be an **increase** in **proteinuria**. This woman is in **renal failure**. Abdominal pain – there is <u>upper</u> abdominal pain. This is due to **liver oedema**. The woman may also have **nausea** and **vomiting**.

16. c. 17. b. 18. c.

19. i: a, b, e, f, g, i, j   ii: c, d, g, l, m   iii: h, k

20. i–b ii–m iii–h iv–f v–i vi–e vii–g viii–d ix–j

21. **a.** Monozygotic twins develop from the fusion of <u>one oocyte and one spermatozoon, which splits in two after fertilization.</u>

b. Dizygotic twins develop from <u>two separate oocytes that are fertilized by two separate spermatozoa.</u>

c. Superfecundation is the term used when twins are conceived from <u>sperm from different men if a woman has had more than one partner during a menstrual cycle.</u>

d. Superfetation is the term used for twins conceived as a result of <u>two coital acts in different menstrual cycles.</u>

e. Zygosity means determining whether or not twins <u>are monozygotic or dizygotic.</u>

22. **a.** Monozygote twins – same sex, same genes, same blood group and physical features, e.g. eyes and hair colour, ear shapes and palm creases – (identical twins).

b. Dizygote twins – alike as brother and sister, can be the same or different sexes – (non-identical twins).

23. True: a, c, d, e, g

    False: b, f

24. c. 25. b. 26. e. 27. d.

1. **Latent first stage:**

   b. The period of time is not necessarily continuous when there are painful contractions.

   c. There is some cervical change, including cervical effacement and dilatation up to 4 cm.

   Established first stage of labour:

   d. There is progressive cervical dilatation from 4 cm.

   h. There are regular painful contractions.

   Passive second stage:

   f. There is a finding of full dilatation of the cervix prior to involuntary expulsive contractions.

   Active second stage:

   a. There is active maternal effort following confirmation of full dilatation of the cervix in the absence of expulsive contractions.

   e. There are expulsive contractions with a finding of full dilatation of the cervix.

   g. The baby is visible.

2. i–c ii–k iii–h iv–i v–j vi–d vii–a viii–l
   ix–e x–f xi–b xii–g

3.

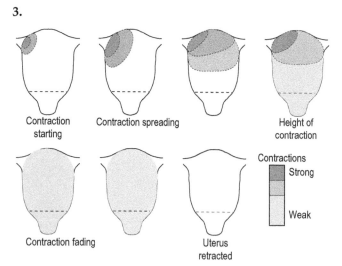

Contraction starting

Contraction spreading

Height of contraction

Contractions

Strong

Weak

Contraction fading

Uterus retracted

Figure 11.1

4. **a.** To assess <u>progress</u> or <u>delay</u> in labour.

   b. To confirm the <u>full dilatation</u> of the <u>cervix</u>.

   c. To make a positive identification of <u>presentation.</u>

   d. To determine whether the (head) is <u>engaged</u> (in case of doubt).

   e. To ascertain whether the <u>forewaters</u> have <u>ruptured</u>, or to <u>rupture</u> them artificially.

   f. To exclude <u>cord prolapse</u> after <u>rupture</u> of the <u>forewaters</u> especially if there is an <u>ill-fitting presenting</u> part or the <u>fetal heart</u> rate changes.

   g. In multiple pregnancy: To confirm the <u>axis</u> of the fetus and <u>presentation</u> of the second <u>twin</u> and, if necessary, in order to <u>rupture</u> the second <u>amniotic sac.</u>

5. **a.** i. Labia for any sign of <u>varicosities, oedema or vulval warts or sores.</u> ii. Perineum for any <u>scars from previous episiotomy or tear including scarring from cultural female genital mutilation.</u> iii. Vaginal orifice: <u>discharge, bleeding.</u> iv. Other observations (if present): <u>Colour and odour of any discharge or amniotic fluid if membranes have ruptured.</u>

   b. i. Rectum – <u>loaded.</u> ii. (In multiparous women) – <u>cystocele.</u>

   c. <u>Effacement</u> and <u>dilatation.</u> <u>Length</u> of the <u>cervical</u> canal, <u>consistency</u> of cervix and <u>application</u> to the presenting part.

   d. i. <u>Present</u> or <u>absent.</u> ii. <u>Intact membranes, consistency of membranes, bulging, ease or difficulty in feeling membranes.</u>

   e. i. <u>Descent</u> – estimation in relationship to maternal <u>ischial spines</u> noting the distance <u>above</u> or <u>below</u> the <u>spines.</u> ii. The presence of <u>moulding</u> or <u>caput succedaneum.</u>

   f. i. The position of the <u>fetal head</u> as defined by the <u>occiput</u> including <u>flexion</u> (using any <u>sutures</u> and <u>fontanelles</u> located).

   g. i. Noting changes in the <u>position</u> of the fetus from a previous assessment.

6. a. Acceleration – This is a brief <u>rise</u> in the fetal heart rate of at least <u>15</u> beats, for at least <u>15</u> s.

b. Deceleration – This is a <u>drop</u> in the fetal heart rate from the <u>baseline</u> of <u>15</u> beats for >15 s but <u><3</u> min.

c. Bradycardia – This is a <u>deceleration</u> of the fetal heart rate lasting longer than <u>3</u> min.

d. Baseline rate - Baseline rate should <u>vary</u> by at least <u>5</u> beats over a period of <u>1</u> min.

7.

		Categorization of Fetal heart rate (FHR) features			
	Feature	Baseline (bpm)	Variability (bpm)	Decelerations	Accelerations
E F M	a. Reassuring	110–160	≥5	<u>None</u>	<u>Present</u>
	b. Non-reassuring	100–109 161–180	<u><5</u> for <u>40–90</u> minutes	Typical variable decelerations with over 50% of contractions occurring for over 90 minutes. Single prolonged deceleration for up to 3 minutes.	The absence of accelerations with an otherwise normal CTG is of uncertain significance
	c. Abnormal	<u><100</u> <u>>180</u> <u>Sinusoidal</u> pattern for ≥10 minutes	<u><5</u> for <u>90</u> minutes	Either atypical variable decelerations with over 50% of contractions or late deceleration, both for over 30 minutes. Single <u>prolonged</u> deceleration <u>>3 minutes.</u>	

8. a. Normal – A FHR trace in which <u>all four features</u> are classified as reassuring.

b. Suspicious – A FHR trace with one feature classified as non-reassuring and the remaining features classified as reassuring.

c. Pathological – A FHR trace with two or more features classified as non-reassuring or one or more classified as abnormal.

9. Pain of labour is associated with an **increased** respiratory rate. This may cause a **decrease** in $PaCO_2$ level with a corresponding **increase** in pH. The fetus is then affected and a subsequent **drop** in the fetal $PaCO_2$ ensues. This may be suspected by the presence of **late** decelerations on the CTG. The acid–base equilibrium of the system may be altered by **hyper**ventilation. **Alkalosis** may then affect the diffusion of **oxygen** across the placenta, leading to a degree of fetal hypoxia.

Cardiac output **increases** by **20%** in first stage and **50%** in second stage of labour. Pain apprehension and fear may cause a **sympathetic** response thereby producing more of an **increase** in cardiac output.

10.

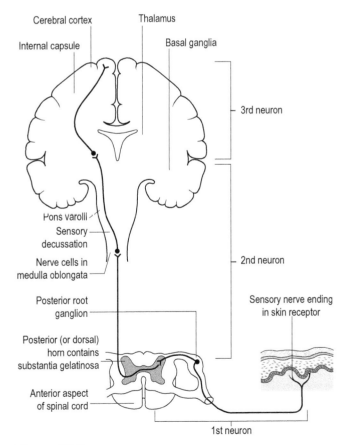

Figure 11.2

11.

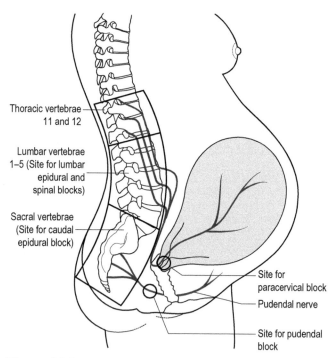

Figure 11.3

12.

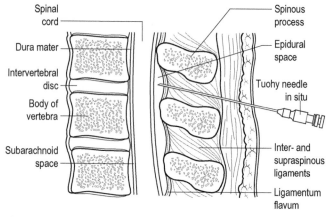

Figure 11.4

13. True: b, c, e, f, g, i

False: a, d, h

14. b.   **15.** c.   **16.** a.   **17.** c.   **18.** a.   **19.** a.   **20.** d.

21. The second stage begins when the cervix is fully dilated. In physiological labour the woman usually feels the urge to expel the fetus. It is complete when the baby is born.

22. a. Fetal axis pressure – This occurs during contractions: the uterus rises forward and the force of the fundal contraction is transmitted to the upper pole of the fetus, down the long axis of the fetus and applied by the presenting part to the cervix.

b. 'Purple line' – This is a pigmented mark in the cleft of the buttocks which creeps up the cleft as labour progresses. It is also called the 'anal cleft line'.

c. Rhomboid of Michaelis – This presents as a dome shaped curve in the lower back, and is held to indicate the posterior displacement of the sacrum and coccyx as the fetal occiput moves into the maternal sacrum.

d. 'Ferguson's reflex' – This phenomenon occurs when pressure from the presenting part stimulates nerve receptors in the pelvic floor. The woman experiences the need to push and this becomes increasingly, compulsive, overwhelming and involuntary. Maternal response is to employ secondary powers of expulsion by contracting her abdominal muscles and diaphragm.

23. a. Anteriorly, the bladder is pushed upwards into the abdomen.

b. The urethra is stretched and thins out so that the lumen is reduced.

c. Posteriorly, the rectum becomes flattened into the sacral curve.

d. The levator ani muscles dilate, thin out and are displaced laterally.

e. The perineal body is flattened, stretched and thinned.

24. Upright positions: squatting, all fours, standing, kneeling, using a birthing ball.

25. Reduced severe pain levels and subsequent responses; less risk of: supine hypotension, reduced placental perfusion, dimished fetal oxygenation, decrease in the efficiency of uterine contractions.

26. a. Descent takes place.

b. Whichever part leads and first meets the resistance of the pelvic floor will rotate forward until it comes under the symphysis pubis

c. Whatever emerges from the pelvis will pivot around the pubic bone.

27. **a.** longitudinal **b.** cephalic **c.** right or left occipitoanterior **d.** good flexion **e.** denominator **f.** posterior part of the anterior parietal bone.

28. Descent → Flexion → Internal rotation of the head → Extension of the head → Restitution → Internal rotation of the shoulders → Lateral flexion.

29. **a.** flexion **b.** restitution **c.** descent **d.** internal rotation of the head **e.** internal rotation of the head **f.** internal rotation of the head **g.** flexion **h.** extension of the head **i.** lateral flexion **j.** extension of the head **k.** internal rotation of the head **l.** restitution **m.** internal rotation of the shoulders

30. **a.** 1-degree – Involves <u>fourchette</u> only.

   b. 2-degree – Involves the <u>fourchette</u> and the <u>superficial perineal</u> muscles, namely the <u>transverse perineal</u> muscles and in some cases the <u>pubococcygeus</u>.

   c. 3-degree – Comprises a <u>partial</u> or <u>complete</u> disruption of the <u>anal sphincter</u> muscles, which may involve either or both <u>external</u> and <u>internal anal sphincter</u> muscles.

   d. 4-degree – Involves a disruption of the <u>anal sphincter</u> muscles with a breach of the <u>rectal mucosa</u>.

31. An episiotomy is an <u>incision through the perineal tissues which is designed to enlarge the vulval outlet during birth</u>.

32. **a.** Mediolateral **b.** Median

33. True: b, c, d, e, f, g

   False: a

34. b. **35.** a. **36.** c. **37.** d.

12 Third stage of labour

ANSWERS

1. a. Third stage – This is the period from the <u>birth of the baby to complete expulsion of the placenta and membranes, involving the separation, descent and expulsion of the placenta and membranes and control of haemorrhage from the placenta site.</u>

b. Duration – Active management of the third stage of labour is diagnosed as prolonged if not completed within <u>30</u> minutes of the birth of the baby (NICE 2007).

Physiological management of the third stage of labour is diagnosed as prolonged if not completed within <u>60</u> minutes of the birth of the baby (NICE 2007).

2.

a. During second stage, the uterine cavity progressively empties, enabling the <u>retraction</u> process to <u>accelerate</u>. At the beginning of third stage, the <u>placental site</u> has already <u>diminished</u> in area by about <u>75</u>%.

↓

b. As this occurs, the placenta becomes <u>compressed</u> and the blood in the <u>intervillous spaces</u> is forced back into the <u>spongy</u> layer of the <u>decidua basalis</u>. <u>Retraction</u> of the <u>oblique</u> uterine muscle fibres exerts pressure on the blood vessels so that blood does not drain back into the maternal system. The vessels during this process are termed '<u>tortuous</u>' as they become tense and <u>congested</u> with blood.

↓

c. With the next contraction, the <u>distended</u> veins burst and a small amount of blood seeps in between the septa of the <u>spongy</u> layer and the <u>placental</u> surface, stripping it from its <u>attachment</u>. As the surface for attachment <u>reduces</u>, the relatively <u>non-elastic</u> placenta begins to <u>detach</u> from the uterine wall.

↓

d. Once separation has occurred, the uterus <u>contracts</u> strongly, <u>forcing</u> placenta and <u>membranes</u> to fall into the <u>lower uterine segment</u> and finally into the <u>vagina</u>.

3.

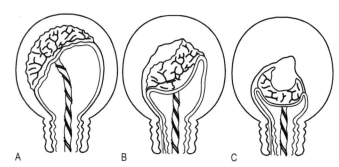

A B C

Figure 12.1 The mechanism of placental separation. (A) Uterine wall is partially retracted, but not sufficiently to cause placental separation. (B) Further contraction and retraction thicken the uterine wall, reduce the placental site and aid placental separation. (C) Complete separation and formation of the retroplacental clot. *Note*: The thin lower segment has collapsed like a concertina following the birth of the baby.

4. a. and **b.**

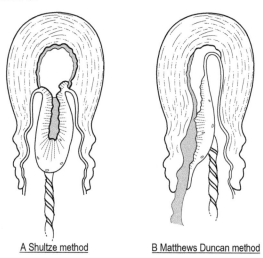

A Shultze method   B Matthews Duncan method

Figure 12.2

c. Method A: a. Schultze; b. Centrally; c. **Yes**; d. Fetal; e. **Shorter**; f. **Less**; g. Complete membranes, retroplacental clot enclosed within membranes.

Method B: a. Matthews Duncan; b. Laterally (one of the borders); c. **No**; d. Maternal; e. **Longer**; f. **More**; g. Ragged membranes, no retroplacental clot.

5. The normal volume of blood flow through a healthy placental site is **500–800** mL/min. Serious haemorrhage would occur at the time of placental separation if blood flow was not arrested within **seconds**. An interplay of the following three factors to control bleeding within the normal physiological processes is essential during this stage:

a. The **tortuous** blood vessels **intertwine through** the **oblique** uterine muscle fibres. **Retraction** of the **oblique** uterine muscle fibres in the **upper** uterine segment results in **thickening** of the muscles. This exerts pressure on the torn vessels, acting as clamps so securing a ligature action.

b. Presence of **vigorous** uterine contraction following separation brings the **uterine** walls into apposition so that **further** pressure is exerted on the **placental site**.

c. Haemostasis is achieved by a transitory **activation** of the coagulation and fibrinolytic systems during, and immediately following, placental separation. This protective response is especially **active** at the placental site so that clot formation in the **torn** vessels is **intensified**. Following separation, the placental site is **rapidly** covered by a **fibrin** mesh utilizing **5–10%** of circulating **fibrinogen**.

6. Ergometrine: c, f, g   Oxytocin: a, b, d, e

7. a. The commonly used brand name of oxytocin is <u>syntocinon</u>.

b. The commonly used brand name of the combined drug ergometrine and oxytocin is <u>syntometrine</u>.

c. The combined action of oxytocin and ergometrine results in a <u>rapid uterine contraction enhanced by a stronger, more sustained contraction lasting several hours</u>.

d. At birth, the timing of administration of a uterotonic drug is usually as the <u>anterior shoulder of the baby is born</u>.

e. The side-effects of the combined drug include <u>elevation of blood pressure</u> and <u>vomiting</u>.

8. a. i. The routine administration of a uterotonic drug (im, iv, or orally)

ii. Cord clamping of the umbilical cord shortly after delivery of the placenta

iii. The use of controlled cord traction (CTT)

b. i. Uterotonic drugs are withheld

ii. The umbilical cord is left unclamped until cord pulsation has ceased.

iii. The placenta is expelled by use of gravity and maternal effort

9. There is a small fresh blood loss, the umbilical cord lengthens, the fundus becomes rounder, smaller and more mobile, the fundus rises in the abdomen above the level of the placenta, the placenta is visible at the vagina.

10. True: b, c, f, h

False: a, d, e, g

11. a. Primary post partum haemorrhage (PPH) – This relates to <u>excessive</u> bleeding from the <u>genital tract at any time following the baby's birth up to 24 hours following birth</u>.

b. Blood loss – Irrespective of maternal condition, blood loss reaching <u>500</u> mL must be treated as a PPH.

c. Secondary postpartum haemorrhage – This relates to any <u>abnormal</u> or <u>excessive</u> bleeding from the <u>genital tract</u> occurring between <u>24 hours</u> and <u>12 weeks</u> postnatally.

12. Atonic uterus, retained placenta, trauma, and blood coagulation disorder.

13. a. An atonic uterus relates to the failure of the <u>myometrium</u> at <u>placental site</u> to <u>contract</u> and <u>retract</u> and to <u>compress</u> torn blood vessels and <u>control</u> blood loss by a <u>living ligature</u> action.

b. i. Pregnancy related: <u>multiple pregnancy</u> or <u>polyhydramnios</u> causing overdistension of the uterine muscle.

ii. Placenta related: Placenta <u>praevia</u> as it partly or wholly lies in the <u>lower segment</u> where the <u>thinner</u> muscle layer contains few <u>oblique</u> fibres resulting in poor control of bleeding. Placenta <u>abruption</u> as blood may have seeped between the <u>muscle</u> fibres interfering with <u>effective</u> muscle action. A severe case results in a <u>Couvelaire</u> uterus.

iii. Labour related: <u>Precipitate</u> labour and <u>prolonged</u> labour resulting in uterine inertia resulting from maternal exhaustion/ sluggishness.

iv. Placental separation: <u>Incomplete, retained placental fragments/membranes and cotyledon.</u>

v. Maternal reasons: <u>Full bladder</u> may be a mechanical reason that interferes with uterine action.

vi. Other: <u>General anaesthesia,</u> which may cause uterine <u>relaxation,</u> e.g. halothane.

14. Previous history of PPH or retained placenta; high parity; fibroids; anaemia; ketosis; HIV/AIDS.

15.

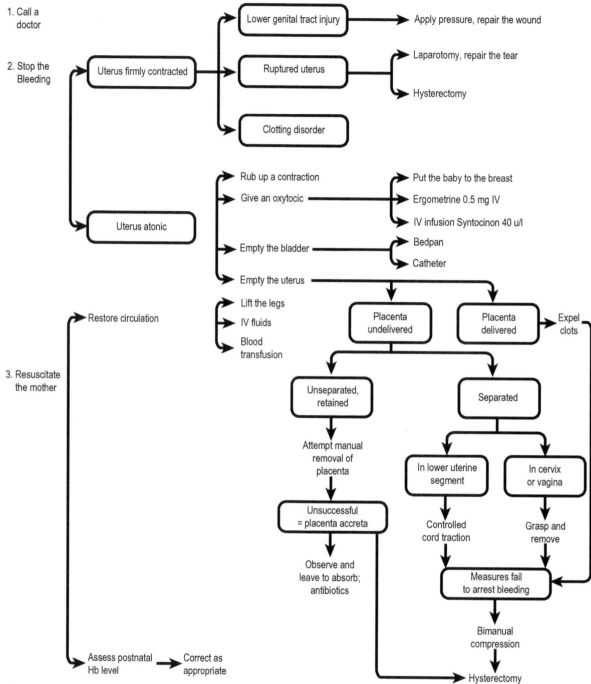

Figure 12.3

16. The fingers of one hand are inserted into the vagina like a **cone**; the hand is formed into a **fist** and placed into the **anterior** vaginal **fornix**, the **elbow** resting on the bed. The other hand is placed behind the uterus **abdominally**, the fingers pointing **towards** the cervix. The **uterus** is brought **forwards** and compressed between the **palm** of the hand positioned **abdominally** and the **fist** in the vagina.

17. True: a, d, e, f

False: b, c

ANSWERS

1. a. 24 weeks   **b.** Women with uncomplicated pregnancies should usually be offered induction of labour between 41+0 and 42+0 weeks to avoid the risks of prolonged pregnancy (NICE 2008). **c.** 24 weeks   **d.** 8   **e.** 1 hour or less

2. True: a, b, c, d, e, g

False: f, h

3.

Inducibility features	0	1	2	3
Dilatation of the cervix (cm)	<1	1–2	2–4	> 4
Consistency of the cervix	Firm	Firm	Med	Soft
Cervical canal length (cm)	>4	2–4	1–2	<1
Position of the cervix	Post	Mid	Ant	N/A
Station of presenting part (cm above or below ischial spines)	-3	-2	-1,0	+1, +2

4. True: b, c, d, e, f, g

False: a, h

5. a.

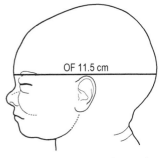

Figure 13.1 Engaging diameter of a deflexed head: occipitofrontal (OF) 11.5 cm.

OF 11.5 cm

b.

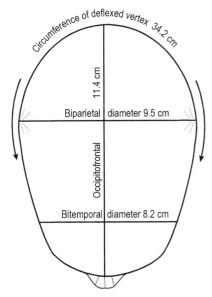

Circumference of deflexed vertex 34.2 cm

11.4 cm

Occipitofrontal

Biparietal diameter 9.5 cm

Bitemporal diameter 8.2 cm

Figure 13.2 Presenting dimensions of a deflexed head.

6. a. The lie is <u>longitudinal</u>.

b. The attitude of the head is <u>deflexed</u>.

c. The presentation is <u>vertex</u>.

d. The position is <u>right</u> occipito<u>posterior</u>.

e. The <u>denominator</u> is the occiput.

f. The presenting part is <u>the middle part or anterior area of the left parietal bone.</u>

g. The <u>occipitofrontal</u> diameter (<u>11.5</u> cm) lies in the right <u>oblique</u> diameter of the pelvic brim. The occiput points to the right sacroiliac joint and the sinciput to the left <u>iliopectineal eminence</u>.

7. Table 13.5A **a.** Descent and flexion (Figure 13.3): <u>Descent</u> takes place with increasing <u>flexion</u>. <u>Sagittal</u> suture lies in the right <u>oblique</u> diameter of the pelvis. The <u>occiput</u> becomes the leading part.

b. Internal rotation of the head (b, c & d) (Figure 13.4): The <u>occiput</u> and shoulders have rotated 1/8th of a circle forwards. Sagittal suture lies in the transverse diameter of the pelvis.

c. (Figure 13.5) The occiput and shoulders have rotated 2/8^ths of a circle forwards. Sagittal suture now lies in the left oblique diameter of the pelvis. The position is right occipitoanterior.

d. (Figure 13.6) The occiput has rotated 3/8^ths of a circle forwards to lie under the symphysis pubis. There is a twist in the neck. Sagittal suture lies in the anteroposterior diameter of the pelvis.

Table 13.5B **e.** Crowning: The occiput escapes under the symphysis pubis.

f. Extension: The sinciput, face, and chin sweep the perineum and the head is born by a movement of extension. **g.** Restitution: The occiput turns 1/8th of a circle to the right and the head realigns with the shoulders. **h.** Internal rotation of the shoulders: The shoulders enter the pelvis in the right oblique diameter; the anterior shoulder reaches the pelvic

floor first and rotates 1/8th of a circle to lie under the symphysis pubis.

i. External rotation of the head: At the same time the occiput turns a further 1/8th of a circle to the right.

j. Lateral flexion: The anterior shoulder escapes under the symphysis pubis, the posterior shoulder sweeps the perineum and the body is born by lateral flexion.

8. In Figure 13.7 the position is **right** occipitoposterior. The occiput fails to rotate forwards in the situation. Instead the **sinciput** reaches the pelvic floor first and rotates **forwards**. The **occiput** goes into the hollow of the sacrum. In Figure 13.8 the position is now direct occipitoposterior. The baby is born facing the pubic bone. This is termed a 'face to pubes' birth.

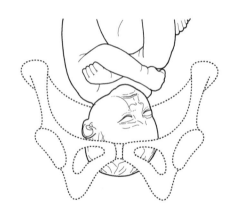

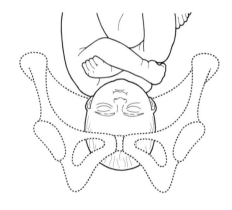

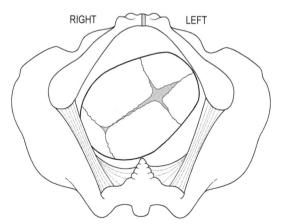

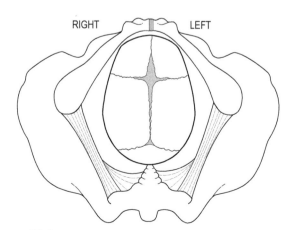

Figure 13.7 Persistent occipitoposterior position before rotation of the occiput: position right occipitoposterior.

Figure 13.8 Persistent occipitoposterior position after short rotation: position direct occipitoposterior.

9. Face presentation: b, e, h   Brow presentation: a, d, f, i   Breech presentation: c, g, j

10.

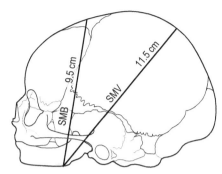

Figure 13.9 Diameters involved in delivery of face presentation. Engaging diameter, sub-mentobregmatic (SMB) 9.5 cm. The sub-mentovertical (SMV) diameter, 11.5 cm, sweeps the perineum.

11. a. The lie is <u>longitudinal.</u>

b. The attitude is one of <u>extension</u> of the <u>head and neck.</u>

c. The presentation is <u>face.</u>

d. The position is <u>left mentoanterior.</u>

e. The denominator is the <u>mentum.</u>

f. The presenting part is the <u>left malar bone.</u>

12.

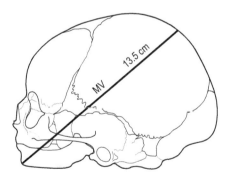

Figure 13.10 Brow presentation. The mentovertical (MV) diameter, 13.5 cm, lies at the pelvic brim.

13. a.

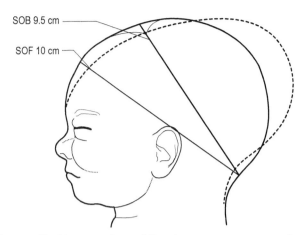

Figure 13.11 Type of moulding in a vertex presentation (SOB, suboccipitobregmatic; SOF, suboccipitofrontal).

b.

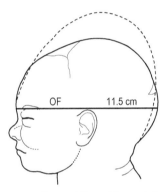

Figure 13.12 Upward moulding (dotted line) following persistent occipitoposterior position. OF, occipitofrontal.

c.

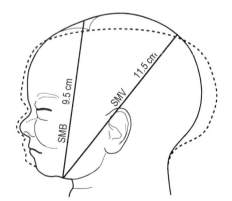

Figure 13.13 Moulding in a face presentation (dotted line). SMB, sub-mentobregmatic; SMV, sub-mentovertical.

d.

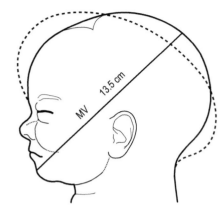

Figure 13.14 Moulding in a brow presentation (dotted line). MV, mentovertical.

14.

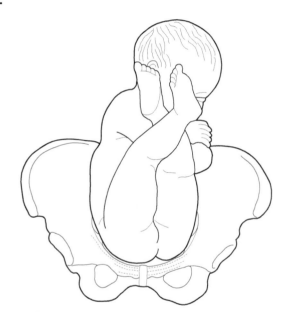

Figure 13.15 Frank breech.

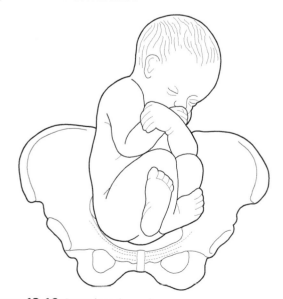

Figure 13.16 Complete breech.

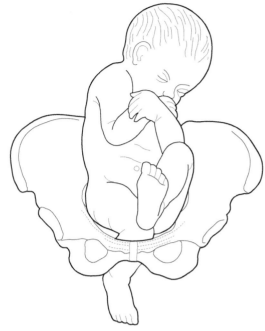

Figure 13.17 Footling presentation.

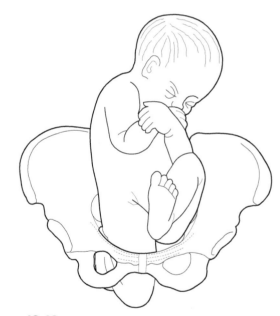

Figure 13.18 Knee presentation.

   a. Frank breech   **b.** Complete breech

   c. Footling breech   **d.** Knee presentation

15. **a.** The lie is <u>longitudinal</u>.

   b. The attitude is on of complete <u>flexion</u>.

   c. The presentation is <u>breech</u>.

   d. The position is <u>left sacroanterior</u>.

   e. The <u>denominator</u> is the sacrum.

   f. The presenting part is the <u>anterior left buttock</u>.

g. The bitrochanteric diameter (10.0 cm) enters the pelvis in the left oblique diameter of the brim. The sacrum points to the iliopectineal eminence.

16. a. On birth of the shoulders the baby is allowed to hang from the vulva **without** support. The baby's weight brings the head onto the pelvic floor on which the occiput rotates. The **sagittal** suture is now in the anteroposterior diameter of the outlet. If the head does not **rotate** then two fingers should be placed on the malar bones and the head rotated. The baby can hang for up to 1 or 2 minutes. Gradually the neck elongates, the hair-line appears and the suboccipital region can be felt. Three methods used to achieve a controlled birth include: i. forceps applied to the after-coming head; ii. Burns Marshall method and iii. Mauriceau-Smellie-Veit manoeuvre. Assistance is required for babies born with extended legs and extended arms. Controlled birth of the head is vital to avoid any sudden change in intracranial pressure.

b. i. This method is conducted once the nape of the neck and hairline are visible.

ii. (A) in Figure 13.19. The baby is grasped by the **feet** and held **on stretch**.

iii. (B) in Figure 13.19. The mouth and nose are free. The vault of the head is delivered **slowly**.

iv. The method involves the attendant standing facing **away from** the mother. With the left hand, the attendant grasps the baby's ankles from behind with the forefinger between the two. The baby is kept on the stretch with sufficient **traction** to prevent the neck from bending backwards and being fractured. The suboccipital region, and not the neck, should pivot under the apex of the **pubic arch** or the spinal cord may be crushed. The feet are taken up through an arc of 180° until the mouth and nose are free at the vulva.

c. i. Mauriceau-Smellie-Veit manoevre is mainly used when there is delay in descent of the head because of **extension**. The manoeuvre promotes jaw **flexion** and shoulder **traction**.

ii. (A) in Figure 13.20. The hands are in position **before** the body is lifted.

iii. (B) in Figure 13.20. This shows extraction of the head.

iv. The manoeuvre involves the baby being laid astride the **arm** with the palm supporting the **chest**. One finger is placed on each malar bone to flex the head. The middle finger may be used to apply pressure to the chin.

Two fingers of the attendant's other hand are hooked over the shoulders with the middle finger pushing up the occiput to aid flexion. Traction is applied to draw the head out of the vagina and, when the suboccipital region appears, the body is lifted to assist the head to pivot around the symphysis pubis. The vault is delivered **slowly**.

d. i. When the popliteal fossae appear at the vulva, **two** fingers are placed along the length of one thigh with the fingertips **in the fossa**. The leg is swept to the side of the abdomen (**abducting the hip**) and the knee is **flexed** by the pressure on its under surface and the **lower** part of the leg will emerge from the vagina. The process is repeated for the other leg.

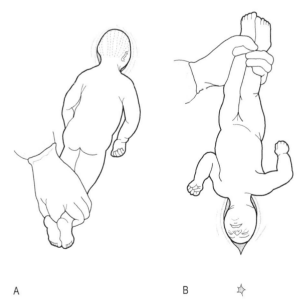

A   B

Figure 13.19 Burns Marshall method of delivering the after-coming head of a breech presentation: (A) The baby is grasped by the feet and held on the stretch. (B) The mouth and nose are free. The vault of the head is delivered slowly.

e.

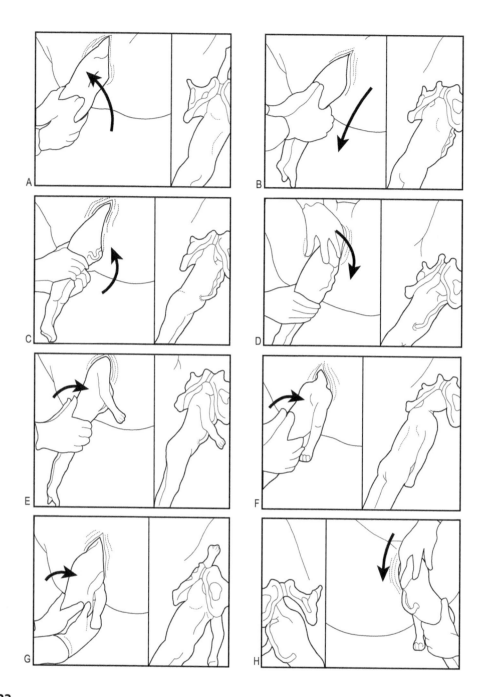

Figure 13.23

f. i. Loveset manoeuvre involves a combination of <u>rotation</u> and **downward** traction to deliver the **arms**. The direction of <u>rotation</u> must always bring the **back** uppermost and the arms are delivered from under the pubic arch. This manoeuvre needs to be conducted promptly to avoid any further delay and possible <u>hypoxia</u>.

Reference

NICE (2008) Induction of labour Guideline. [Online] Available at: http://www.nice.org.uk/guidance/ CG70/NICEGuidance [Accessed 24 April 2012].

17. b.   **18.** b.   **19.** b.   **20.** c.   **21.** c.

CHAPTER 14

Midwifery and obstetric emergencies

ANSWERS

1. True: a, d, f, g, h

   False: b, c, e

2. **a.** Knee-chest position.

   b. Exaggerated Sim's position.

   c. To relieve pressure on the umbilical cord. The fetus will gravitate towards the diaphragm.

   d. Lower the top of the bed (head down) or raise the foot of the bed (Trendelenburg position).

3. **a.** Call for assistance and note the <u>time</u>.

   b. If the cord lies outside the vagina, then it should be gently <u>replaced</u> to prevent <u>spasm</u>, to maintain <u>temperature</u> and prevent <u>drying</u>.

   c. Oxygen may be administered to the mother by face mask at <u>4</u> L/min, which may improve fetal <u>oxygenation</u>.

   d. The midwife may need to keep her <u>fingers</u> in the <u>vagina</u> and hold the <u>presenting part</u> off the umbilical cord, especially during a <u>contraction</u>.

   e. i. Birth will be by <u>caesarean section</u> if the fetus is alive but vaginal birth is not imminent. ii. Birth may be by <u>vaginal birth</u> with the midwife performing an <u>episiotomy</u> if the cord prolapse is diagnosed in second stage (multiparous mother). iii. Where the presentation is cephalic, birth may be assisted and achieved through <u>ventouse</u> or <u>forceps</u>.

4. Shoulder dystocia occurs when the <u>anterior</u> shoulder becomes trapped <u>behind</u> or on the <u>symphysis pubis</u>, while the <u>posterior</u> shoulder may be in the <u>hollow</u> of the <u>sacrum</u> or high above the <u>sacral promontory</u>. In shoulder dystocia, the <u>impaction</u> is at the pelvic <u>inlet</u> and the force of <u>gravity</u> will keep the fetus against the mother's <u>uterus</u> and <u>pelvis</u>.

5. **H**: Call for help. **E**: Episiotomy need assessed. **L**: Legs in McRoberts position. **P**: Pressure suprapubically. **E**: Enter vagina (internal rotation). **R**: Remove posterior arm. **R**: Roll the woman over and try again.

6. **a.** The term 'adduct' means to pull or move something (e.g. arm or leg) **towards** the midline of the body or a toe or finger **towards** the axis of the leg or arm.

   b. The term 'abduct' means to pull or move something (e.g. arm or leg) **away from** the midline of the body or a toe or finger **away from** the axis of the leg or arm.

7. **a.** <u>McRoberts manoeuvre</u>. This manoeuvre will **rotate** the angle of the <u>symphysis pubis</u> superiorly and use the <u>weight</u> of the mother's legs to create gentle <u>pressure</u> on her abdomen, releasing the impaction of the **anterior** shoulder.

   b. Correct application of <u>suprapubic pressure</u>. Pressure should be exerted on the side of the fetal **back** and towards the fetal **chest**. This manoeuvre may help to **adduct** the shoulders and push the **anterior** shoulder away from the <u>symphysis pubis</u> into the larger oblique or transverse diameter.

   c. The 'all fours position' may be especially helpful if the <u>posterior</u> shoulder is impacted behind the <u>sacral promontory</u> as this position optimizes space available in the sacral curve and may allow the <u>posterior</u> shoulder to be delivered first.

8. **a.** <u>Rubin's manoeuvre</u>. In this manoeuvre, the midwife on VE needs to identify the **posterior** shoulder. Then the **posterior** shoulder is pushed in the direction of the fetal **chest**, thus rotating the **anterior** shoulder away from the <u>symphysis pubis</u>. **Adducting** the shoulders reduces the 12 cm bisacromial diameter.

   b. <u>Woods' manoeuvre</u>. In this manoeuvre, the midwife inserts her hand into the vagina and identifies the fetal **chest**. Pressure is exerted on the **posterior** fetal shoulder achieving rotation. This manoeuvre **abducts** the shoulders and also rotates the shoulders into a more favourable diameter for birth.

c. Delivery of the posterior arm: This manoeuvre makes use of the space created by the <u>hollow</u> of the <u>sacrum</u> (as seen in A and B). Figure C shows two fingers splinting the **humerus** of the **posterior** arm. Figure D shows the elbow **flexed** and the forearm being swept over the **chest** to deliver the hand.

9. a–ii b–ii and iii c–iii d–i e–i

10. a–iv b–ii c–v d–i e–vi f–iii

11. a–iii b–ii c–iv d–i e – iv f–i g–iv

12.

Skin → fat → rectus sheath

    → muscle (rectus abdominis) → abdominal peritoneum

    → pelvic peritoneum → uterine muscle

13. a–v b–iii c–i d–ii e–iv

14. Shock is a <u>complex</u> syndrome involving a <u>reduction</u> in blood flow to the <u>tissues</u> that may result in irreversible <u>organ</u> damage and progressive <u>collapse</u> of the <u>circulatory</u> system. If left untreated it will result in <u>death</u>.

Shock can be <u>acute</u> but prompt treatment results in <u>recovery</u> with little detrimental effect on the mother. However <u>inadequate</u> treatment or <u>failure</u> to initiate effective treatment can result in a <u>chronic</u> condition ending in <u>multisystem</u> organ failure which may be <u>fatal</u>.

15. a. Severe obstetric haemorrhage (APH – vasa praevia, placenta praevia PPH).

b. Allergy to peanuts, penicillin or other drug.

c. Acute uterine inversion.

d. Overwhelming infection general or associated with pregnancy and childbirth, e.g. infection entering through the placenta (most common potentially fatal is beta haemolytic *Streptococcus pyogenes*).

e. Pulmonary embolism or women with cardiac defects.

16. a. The **drop** in cardiac output produces a response from the **sympathetic** nervous system through the activation of receptors in the **aorta and carotid arteries**. Blood is redistributed to the **vital organs**. There is **constriction** of the vessel in the gastrointestinal tract, kidneys, skin, and lungs. Peristalsis **slows**, urinary output is **reduced** and exchange of gas is impaired as blood flow **diminishes**. The heart rate **increases** and the pupils of the eyes **dilate**. Sweat glands are **stimulated** and the skin becomes **moist and clammy**. Adrenaline (Epinephrine) is released from the adrenal **medulla** and aldosterone from the adrenal **cortex**. Antidiuretic hormone (ADH) is secreted from the **posterior** lobe of the pituitary gland. Their combined effect is to cause **vasoconstriction, increased** cardiac output and a **decrease** in urinary output. Venous return to the heart will **increase** but this will not be sustained unless the fluid loss is replaced.

b. Gas exchange is **impaired** as the physiological dead space **increases** within the lungs. Levels of carbon dioxide **rise** and arterial oxygen levels **fall**. **Ischaemia** within the lungs alters the production of **surfactant** and as a result of this, alveoli **collapse**. Oedema in the lungs, due to **increased** permeability, **exacerbates** the existing problem of diffusion of oxygen. Atelectasis, oedema and **reduced** compliance impair ventilation and gaseous exchange, leading ultimately to respiratory **failure**.

17. Amniotic fluid embolism occurs when amniotic fluid enters the **maternal** circulation via the <u>uterus</u> or <u>placental</u> site. Maternal collapse can be **rapidly** progressive. The body's initial response is pulmonary **vasospasm** causing hypoxia, **hypotension**, <u>pulmonary</u> oedema and cardiovascular collapse. Secondly there is the development of **left** ventricular failure, with haemorrhage and <u>coagulation</u> disorder and further uncontrollable <u>haemorrhage</u>. There is uterine **hypertonus** and this will induce fetal <u>compromise</u> in response to uterine <u>hypoxia</u>.

18. a. <u>tachycardia</u>; <u>hypotension</u>; <u>pale clammy skin and shivering</u>

b. <u>cyanosis</u>; <u>dyspnoea</u>

c. <u>haemorrhage from the placental site</u>

d. <u>restlessness</u>, <u>panic</u>, <u>abnormal behaviour</u>; <u>convulsions</u>

19. a. Shake and <u>shout</u>.

b. Call for <u>help</u>.

c. A – <u>airway</u>. Check for chest movement.

d. B – <u>breathing</u>. Listen for breaths.

e. C – <u>circulation</u>. Check for pulse.

f. Appropriate position for body: <u>Laid flat on back removing pillows</u>. Precaution for pregnancy: <u>position the woman with a left lateral tilt to prevent aortocaval compression</u>.

g. Position for head: <u>Tilted back and the chin lifted upwards to open airway</u>.

h. Use 30 compressions : 2 breaths (or as per updated resuscitation guidelines).

i. Continue until <u>help arrives</u>.

Always refer to updated resuscitation guidelines.

20.

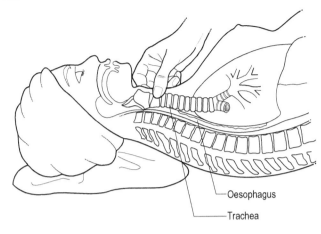

—Oesophagus

—Trachea

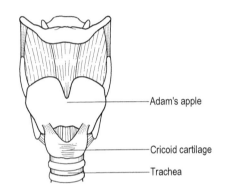

—Adam's apple

—Cricoid cartilage

—Trachea

Figure 14.8

21. c. **22.** d. **23.** d. **24.** d. **25.** a.

15 The puerperium

ANSWERS

1. a. The puerperium starts immediately after delivery of the <u>placenta</u> and <u>membranes</u> and continues for <u>6</u> weeks (in the absence of complications). It is expected that by this time all the <u>body systems</u> will have recovered from the effects of pregnancy and returned to their <u>non-pregnant</u> state.

b. The postnatal period is defined in the UK as <u>a period after the end of labour during which the attendance of a midwife upon a woman and baby is required, being not less than 10 days and for such longer period as the midwife considers necessary</u> (NMC 2004).

c. i. <u>Oestrogen</u>. ii. <u>Progesterone</u>. iii. <u>Human chorionic gonadotrophin</u> iv. <u>Human placental lactogen</u>.

2. On expulsion of the placenta and membranes, the muscle layers of the <u>myometrium</u> simulate the action of <u>ligatures</u> that compress and occlude the large <u>sinuses</u> of the blood vessels exposed by placental separation to reduce <u>blood loss</u>. In addition, de-oxygenation and a state of <u>ischaemia</u> arise in tissues due to <u>vasoconstriction</u> in the overall blood supply to the uterus. Through the process of <u>autolysis</u>, autodigestion of the <u>ischaemic</u> muscle fibres by <u>proteolytic</u> enzymes occurs resulting in an overall <u>reduction</u> in their size. There is <u>phagocytic</u> action of polymorphs and <u>macrophages</u> in the blood and lymphatic systems upon the waste products of autolysis, which are then excreted via the <u>renal</u> system in the urine. <u>Coagulation</u> takes place through platelet aggregation and the release of <u>thromboplastin</u> and fibrin.

Apart from the placental site, what remains of the inner surface of the uterine lining, regenerates rapidly to produce a covering of <u>epithelium</u>. Partial covering occurs within <u>7–10</u> days after birth; total coverage is complete by the <u>21st</u> day. Once the placenta has separated, there is a <u>reduction</u> in the circulating levels of hormones related to pregnancy. This leads to further physiological changes in muscle and connective tissue as well as having a major influence on the secretion of <u>prolactin</u> from the <u>anterior</u> pituitary gland.

On initial abdominal palpation the fundus of the uterus should be located <u>centrally</u>, its position being at the same level or slightly <u>below</u> the umbilicus and should feel <u>firm</u> to confirm it is in a state of <u>contraction</u>.

3. a. On palpation the uterus may be <u>poorly</u> contracted and feel wide and 'boggy'. This might be described as 'sub-<u>involution</u>'.

The fundus may be <u>deviated</u> to one side and not progressively <u>reducing</u> in size.

The woman may experience <u>tenderness</u> on palpation.

When compared with findings from a previous examination, <u>blood</u> loss may be fresher and <u>heavier</u> or <u>scanty</u> but <u>foul</u> smelling.

The woman may pass <u>clots</u>.

b. There may be:

<u>Inflammation</u> and tenderness around a wound area.

<u>Slow</u> healing or <u>gaping</u> at the skin edges.

<u>Pain</u> felt deeper in the wound area (as experienced by the woman).

Virulent clear or <u>purulent</u> exudate.

c. Breasts - May feel tight and <u>swollen</u>.

One segment may be flushed or <u>inflamed</u>.

One or both nipples may have <u>cracked</u>, broken or/ discoloured/flaky skin.

4. True: b, c, d, e, f

False: a, g

5.

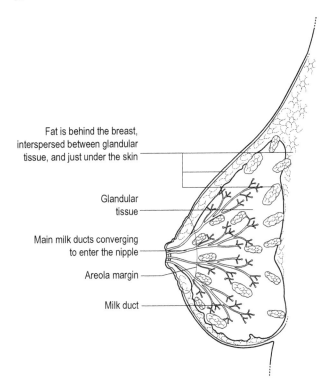

Fat is behind the breast, interspersed between glandular tissue, and just under the skin

Glandular tissue

Main milk ducts converging to enter the nipple

Areola margin

Milk duct

Figure 15.1

6. The alveoli contain <u>acini</u> cells, which produce milk and are surrounded by <u>myoepithelial</u> cells which contract and propel the milk out. Small <u>lactiferous ducts</u>, carrying milk from the alveoli, unite to form larger ducts. Several large ducts (<u>lactiferous tubules</u>) conveying milk from one or more <u>lobe</u> emerge on the surface of the <u>nipple</u>. Myoepithelial cells are orientated <u>longitudinally</u> along the ducts and, under the influence of <u>oxytocin</u>, these smooth muscle cells contract and the tubule becomes <u>shorter</u> and wider. The tubule <u>distends</u> during active milk flow, while the <u>myoepithelial</u> cells are maintained in a state of contracting by circulating <u>oxytocin</u> (2–3 min). The <u>fuller</u> the breast when let down occurs, the greater the degree of <u>ductal</u> distension.

As lactation progresses, the <u>prolactin</u> response to suckling diminishes and <u>milk removal</u> becomes the driving force behind milk production. This is due to <u>whey protein</u> in secreted milk that is able to <u>inhibit</u> the synthesis of milk constituents. This protein accumulates in the breast as the milk <u>accumulates</u> and it exerts <u>negative feedback control</u> on the continued production of milk. Removal of this <u>autocrine inhibitory factor</u> by removing the milk, allows milk production to be <u>stepped up</u> again. This is sometimes referred to as feedback inhibitor of lactation (FIL).

7. True: a, c, d, g, i, j

False: b, e, f, h

8. a. Colostrum has a <u>higher</u> fat and protein content than mature milk.

b. <u>Foremilk</u> (at the beginning of the feed) is of a high volume of relatively <u>low fat</u> milk. <u>Hindmilk</u> (as the feed progresses) <u>decreases</u> in volume with an <u>increase</u> in the proportion of fat sometimes by as much as five times the initial value.

c. It is the <u>fat</u> content and not the <u>protein</u> that has particular significance for the <u>rapidly</u> growing brain of the newborn. The fat content is <u>lowest</u> in the morning and <u>highest</u> in the afternoon.

d. The main carbohydrate component is provided by <u>lactose</u> (which provides the baby with about 40% calorific requirement). This enhances the absorption of <u>calcium</u> and promotes the growth of <u>lactobacilli</u> which <u>increase</u> intestinal acidity thus reducing the growth of pathogenic organisms.

e. The dominant protein is <u>whey</u> which forms soft, flocculent <u>curds</u> when acidified in the stomach.

f. The <u>bifidus factor</u> promotes the growth of Gram-positive bacilli in the gut flora, particularly *Lactobacillus bifidus*, which discourages the multiplication of pathogens. <u>Lactoferrin</u> binds to enteric iron, preventing pathogenic *E. coli* from obtaining the iron needed for them to survive.

g. All the vitamins required for good nutrition and health are supplied in breastmilk. <u>Fat soluble</u> vitamin K is present in milk and is essential for the synthesis of <u>blood-clotting</u> factors. It is present in greater concentrations in <u>colostrum</u> and in the high fat <u>hindmilk</u>.

h. <u>Immunoglobulins</u> are present to provide protection. The most important for the baby is <u>IgA</u> which covers the intestinal epithelium and protects the <u>mucosal</u> surfaces against pathogenic bacteria and enteroviruses.

9. a–iv   b– i   c–viii   d–ii   e–v   f–vi   g–vii   h–iii

10. c.   **11.** c.   **12.** c.   **13.** b.   **14.** e.   **15.** d.   **16.** b.
17. d.   **18.** c.

16 Complementary therapies and pharmacology in childbirth

ANSWERS

1. a. Group 1: 1. Acupuncture; 6. Chiropractic; 9. Herbal medicine; 10. Homeopathy; 19. Oesteopathy.

b. Group 2: 2. Alexander technique; 4. Aromatherapy; 5. Bach flower remedies; 11. Hypnotherapy/hypnosis; 16. Massage; 18. Nutritional therapies; 21. Reflexology/reflex zone therapy; 22. Reiki; 23. Shiatsu; 24. Stress management; 27. Yoga.

c. Group 3a – traditional systems: 3. Anthroposophical medicine; 12. Indian Ayurvedic medicine; 14. Japanese kampo; 17. Naturopathy; 25. Traditional Chinese medicine (TCM); 26. Tibetan medicine. **Group 3b** – diagnostic therapies: 7. Crystal therapies; 8. Dowsing; 13. Iridology; 15. Kinesiology; 20. Radionics.

2. True: a, b, c, e, g, h

False: d, f, i

3. The herb used in this technique is a stick of dried **mugwort**. This is used as a **heat** source over **Bladder** 67 acupuncture point on the **outer** edges of the **little** toes. This is thought to stimulate **adrenocortical** output which causes an **increase** in placental lactogens and changes in **prostaglandins.** Myometrial sensitivity and contractility is **increased**. In turn the fetal heart rate **increases** and there is an **increase** in fetal **movements**. This causes the fetus to turn so that the breech is in the **upper** pole of the uterus and the cephalic to be in the **lower** pole of the uterus. The procedure is normally done around **34–35 weeks'** gestation and performed on **two** feet for **15** min, twice daily for up to **5 days.**

4. From the literature, it is generally thought that the most effective leaves for easing engorgement are the dark green cabbage leaves (only one study has found the white cabbage leaves more effective). This is caused by a chemical in the chlorophyll that

aids the process of drawing off excess fluid. The remedy is based on the process of osmosis. The leaves should be wiped clean and not washed so that it does not interfere with this process. Most women prefer the leaves to be cooled in the refrigerator as a comfort measure. The leaves should be placed inside the brassiere, left until damp and then replaced with new leaves. Repeat the process until relief is obtained.

5. a. Organogenesis occurs between approximately 18 and 55 days post-conception (i.e. 4 and 10 weeks of pregnancy).

b. 'Teratogen' refers to a substance that leads to the birth of a malformed baby if it is present in the body during organogenesis.

c. Factors influencing passage of drugs across the placenta and breast are: i. the size of the molecule, ii. the ionization of the molecule (i.e. +ve or −ve), iii. the lipid or water solubility and iv. the protein binding capacity. In general, molecules of a large size do not cross the placenta and smaller sized molecules cross very easily.

6. a. Prolonged time in the gut. Changes in the **absorption** of oral drugs.

b. Increased circulating plasma volume results in **increased** volume. **Decrease** in the plasma concentration.

c. Increase in blood flow to the kidneys. **Increase** in the rate of excretion of the drug.

d. Increased amounts of total body water and fat. May alter the **distribution** of the drug.

e. Some metabolic pathways in the liver **increase.** **Quicker** metabolism.

f. Major changes in levels of plasma proteins to which some drugs bind. The amount of drug available is **affected.**

7. a–i   b–ii   c–iii   d–v   e–iv

8. a. Cardiac defects   **b.** Facial anomalies, CNS anomalies   **c.** Neural tube defects   **d.** Craniofacial abnormalities   **e.** Craniofacial, cardiac and CNS anomalies.

9. a–v   b–i   c–ii   d–iii   e–iv

10. True: a, c, d, f, h, i

False: b, e, g

11. c.   **12.** b.   **13.** d.   **14.** a.

1. The fetus responds to hypoxia by <u>accelerating</u> the heart rate in an effort to maintain supplies of <u>oxygen</u> to the brain. If hypoxia persists, glucose depletion will stimulate <u>anaerobic glycolysis</u>. This results in a <u>metabolic acidosis</u>. Cerebral <u>vessels</u> will dilate and some brain swelling may occur. <u>Bradycardia</u> develops as the fetus becomes more acidotic and cardiac <u>glycogen reserves</u> are depleted. The anal sphincter <u>relaxes</u> and the fetus may pass <u>meconium</u> into the liquor. Hypoxia triggers <u>gasping</u>, breathing movements which may result in the <u>aspiration</u> of <u>meconium-stained</u> liquor into the lungs.

2.

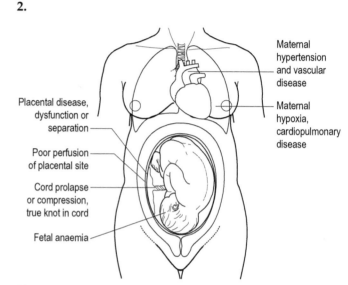

Maternal hypertension and vascular disease

Maternal hypoxia, cardiopulmonary disease

Placental disease, dysfunction or separation

Poor perfusion of placental site

Cord prolapse or compression, true knot in cord

Fetal anaemia

Figure 17.1

3.

Sign	Score		
	0	**1**	**2**
Heart rate	Absent	<100 bpm	>100 bpm
Respiratory effort	Absent	Slow, irregular	Good or crying
Muscle tone	Limp	Some flexion of the limbs	Active
Reflex response to stimuli	None	Minimal grimace	Cough or sneeze
Colour	Blue, pale	Body pink, extremities blue	Completely pink

4. **A: Appearance** (relates to colour); **P: Pulse** (relates to heart rate); **G: Grimace** (relates to response to stimuli); **A: Active** (relates to tone); **R: Respirations** (relates to breathing).

5. **a.** Pulmonary adaptation:

Respiration is stimulated by mild **hypercapnia**, hypoxia and **acidosis**. There is a change in the rhythm of respiration from **episodic shallow** fetal respiration to **regular deeper** breathing. This is due to a combination of chemical and neural stimuli, notably a **fall** in pH level, a **fall** in PaO_2 and a **rise** in $PaCO_2$. Considerable **negative** intrathoracic pressure of up to 9.8 kPa (**100** cm water) is exerted as the first breath is taken. The pressure exerted to

effect **inhalation diminishes** with each breath taken until only **5 cm** of water is required to **inflate** each lung. This is due to surfactant.

b. List other respiratory stimuli: <u>light</u>, <u>noise</u>, <u>touch</u> and pain.

c. Surfactant is a complex of proteins and **lipoproteins**. In utero, the amount of surfactant **increases** until the lungs are mature at **30–34 weeks'** gestation. It is produced by **type 2** epithelial cells in the lungs and lines the **alveoli** to **reduce** the **surface tension** within the **alveoli**. This permits **residual air** to remain in the **alveoli** between breaths and prevent them from **collapsing** at the **end** of each expiration. Surfactant **reduces** the work or effort of breathing.

d. Cardiovascular adaptation:

At birth, the lungs expand and pulmonary vascular resistance is **lowered**. This results in the majority of cardiac output being sent to the lungs.

Oxygenated blood returning to the heart from the lungs **increases** the pressure within the **left** atrium. At the same time, pressure in the **right** atrium is **lowered** because blood ceases to flow through the cord. This brings about functional closure of the **foramen ovale**.

Contraction of the walls of the **ductus arteriosus** occurs almost immediately after birth. This is thought to occur because of the sensitivity of the muscle of the **ductus arteriosus** to **increased** oxygen tension and **reduction** in circulating prostaglandins. There is usually functional closure of the **ductus arteriosus** within **8–10 hours** of birth with complete closure taking place within **several months**.

The remaining temporary structures of the fetal circulation – **umbilical vein**, **ductus venosus** and hypogastric **arteries** – close functionally within a few **minutes** after birth and constriction of the cord. Anatomical closure of fibrous tissue occurs within 2–3 months.

6. Complete the following statements in relation to thermal adaptation by inserting the correct missing words.

a. 37.7°C **b.** 21°C **c.** i. evaporation;
ii. conduction; iii. radiation; iv. convection
d. large, head **e.** thin **f.** shiver **g.** muscle activity

7.

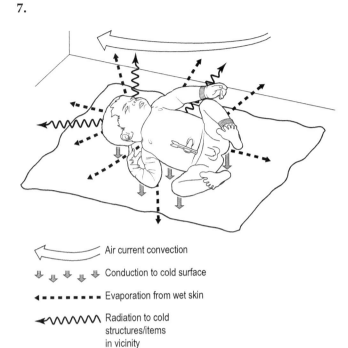

⬳ Air current convection

⬇⬇⬇⬇⬇ Conduction to cold surface

◀- - - - - - - Evaporation from wet skin

◀〜〜〜 Radiation to cold structures/items in vicinity

Figure 17.2

8.

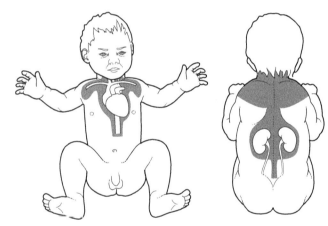

Figure 17.3 Sites of brown fat.

9. Cold stress causes <u>vasoconstriction</u>, thus reducing pulmonary perfusion. Respiratory <u>acidosis</u> develops as the pH and PaO_2 of the blood <u>decrease</u> and the $PaCO_2$ <u>increases</u> leading to respiratory distress exhibited by <u>tachypnoea</u>. This condition is characterized by <u>rapid</u> respirations of up to 120/min. It is common after a caesarean section. The baby may be <u>cyanosed</u> but maintains normal blood gases apart from PaO_2. There is little or no recession of the <u>rib cage</u> and there is minimum, if any, <u>grunt</u> on expiration. The <u>respiratory rate</u> may remain elevated for up to 5 days.

10. a. The baby is <u>dried</u> quickly. The <u>clock timer</u> is started. The <u>radiant heater</u> is switched on to prevent <u>hypothermia.</u> The head should be put in the neutral position to maintain the <u>airway</u> and keep the <u>trachea</u> straightened. If necessary, a small <u>towel</u> can be put under the baby's <u>shoulders</u> to cause slight extension of the <u>head</u>. Review for signs of respiratory effort.

↓

b. If the baby fails to respond then <u>assisted ventilation</u> is necessary.

Place a correctly fitting face mask to cover the <u>nose and mouth</u> and ensures a good seal. Use a 500 mL self-inflating bag to <u>aerate</u> the lungs, deliver five <u>sustained</u> inflations (each breath is for 2–3 seconds). Review for <u>chest movement</u>.

If YES – this is present: continue to <u>ventilate</u> at a rate of <u>40</u> respirations per minute (ventilation breaths).

If NO – this is not present: then review the <u>head</u> position and re-commence the five <u>inflation</u> breaths. Move into <u>ventilation</u> breaths once <u>chest movement</u> has been confirmed.

Outcome: Baby is breathing spontaneously.

11. a. Chest compressions should be performed if the heart rate is < <u>60</u> bpm.

b. The chest is depressed at a rate of <u>100–120</u> times/min, at a ratio of <u>three</u> compressions to <u>one</u> ventilation and at a depth of <u>2–3</u> cm of the baby's chest. N.B. For resuscitation guidance – always refer to the most current resuscitation guidelines.

12. True: a, c, d, e, g

False: b, f, h

13. e.   **14.** a.   **15.** d.   **16.** b.   **17.** b.

1. **a.** 36.5 and 37.3°C

   b. 40 and 60 breaths/min

   c. 110 and 160 beats per min

   d. 13 and 20 g/dL, 50–85%

   e. 24 hours, 48–72 hours

   f. hypothyroidism, cystic fibrosis, phenylketonuria

2. **a.** 2500 g **b.** 1500 g **c.** 1000 g **d.** 37th

3. True: c, d, e, f, g

   False: a, b

4. a–8 b–10 c–2 d–5
   e–11 f–6 g–7 h–9 i–1 j–3 k–13 l–4
   m–14 n–12

5. **a.** Pallor, central cyanosis, jaundice

   b. Apnoea

   c. <110 bpm or >180 bpm (taken during spells of inactivity)

   d. <30 or >60 breaths per min

   e. <36.2°C or > 37.2°C

   f. movement and responsiveness

   g. hypotonic or hypertonic

   h. interest

6. **a.** Cyanosis

   b. tachypnoea

   c. tachycardia

   d. breathless and sweaty during feeds

   e. A sudden gain in weight leading to clinical signs of oedema: this is usually noted in the baby having puffy feet or eyelids and in males, the scrotum may be swollen

   f. systolic

   g. cardiac

   h. liver

7. True: a, c, d, e, h, i

   False: b, f, g

8. a–ii b–iii c–iv d–v e–vi f–i

9. A neutral thermal environment is defined as the ambient air temperature at which oxygen consumption or heat production is minimal, with body temperature in the normal range.

10. **a.** Caput succedaneum refers to a diffuse oedematous swelling under the scalp and above the periosteum. It occurs during labour. It is caused by pressure on the fetal part overlying the cervical os.

    b. Cephalhaematoma refers to an effusion of blood under the periosteum that covers the skull bones. This occurs during vaginal birth. It is due to friction between the fetal skull and maternal pelvic bones resulting in the periosteum being torn from the bone resulting in bleeding.

11.

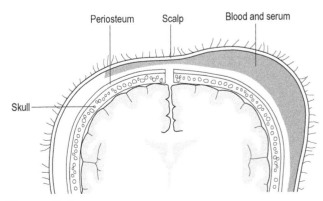

Figure 18.1

12.

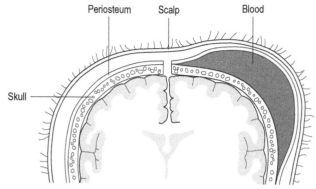

Periosteum   Scalp   Blood

Skull

Figure 18.2

13. Cephalhaematoma: a, c, g, h, j, k, m, o, p, q, r, s

Caput succedaneum: b, d, e, f, i, l, n

14. a–4   b–8   c(i)–1; (ii)–2, 3, 5   d–6   e–7   f–9

15. c.   **16.** c.   **17.** b.   **18.** f.   **19.** a.   **20.** b.

ANSWERS

1. a. Haem is converted to <u>biliverdin</u> and then to <u>unconjugated bilirubin</u>.

b. Globin is broken down into <u>amino acids</u> and used by the body to make <u>proteins</u>.

c. Iron is stored in the <u>body</u> or used for <u>new red cells</u>.

2. a. Unconjugated bilirubin is **fat soluble** and cannot be excreted easily in bile or urine.

b. Conjugated bilirubin has been made **water soluble** in the liver and can be excreted in faeces and urine.

3.

i. Transport of bilirubin:
Unconjugated or <u>fat soluble</u> bilirubin is transported to the liver bound to <u>albumin</u>. If not attached <u>to albumin</u> then this unbound or 'free' <u>bilirubin</u> can be deposited in extravascular <u>fatty</u> and <u>nerve</u> tissues (skin and <u>brain</u>). Skin deposits of unconjugated or <u>fat soluble</u> bilirubin cause jaundice, while <u>brain</u> deposits can cause 'bilirubin <u>toxicity</u>' or kernicterus.

↓

ii. Conjugation:
Once in the liver, unconjugated bilirubin is detached from <u>albumin</u>, combined with <u>glucose</u> and glucoronic acid and conjugation occurs in the presence of <u>oxygen</u> and the <u>enzyme</u> uridine diphosphoglucuronyl transferase (UDP-GT). The conjugated bilirubin is now <u>water-soluble</u> and available for excretion.

↓

iii. Excretion:
Conjugated bilirubin is excreted via the <u>biliary</u> system into the small intestine where normal <u>bacteria</u> change the conjugated bilirubin into <u>urobilinogen</u>. This is then oxidized into orange-coloured <u>urobilin</u>. Most is excreted in the <u>faeces</u> with a small amount excreted in the <u>urine</u>.

4. Neonatal physiological jaundice occurs when unconjugated (<u>fat</u> soluble) bilirubin is deposited in the <u>skin</u> instead of being taken to the <u>liver</u> for processing into conjugated (<u>water</u> soluble) bilirubin that can be excreted in <u>faeces</u> or <u>urine</u>. It is a normal transitional state affecting up to <u>50</u>% of term babies and <u>80</u>% of preterm babies who have a progressive rise in <u>unconjugated</u> bilrubin levels with jaundice on day <u>3</u>.

Physiological jaundice *never* appears before <u>24</u> hours of life and usually fades by <u>1</u> week and bilirubin levels never exceed <u>200–215</u> μmol/L (<u>12–13</u> mg/dL).

5. a–ii b–iv c–ii d–ii e–iii f–i

6. a. Kernicterus (bilirubin toxicity) is an <u>encephalo</u>pathy caused by <u>deposits</u> of <u>unconjugated</u> bilirubin in the <u>basal</u> ganglia of the <u>brain</u>.

b. Early signs can be <u>insidious</u> and include and include (identify as least two): <u>lethargy</u>, <u>changes in muscle tone</u>, <u>a high pitched cry</u> and <u>irritability</u>.

c. Long-term clinical features can include (identify at least four): <u>deafness</u>, <u>blindness</u>, <u>cerebral palsy</u>, <u>developmental delay</u>, <u>learning difficulties</u>, and <u>extrapyramidal disturbances</u> such as <u>athetosis</u>, drooling, <u>facial grimace</u> and <u>chewing</u>, and <u>swallowing difficulties</u>.

7. a. Jaundice usually occurs within the first <u>24</u> hours of life

b. A rapid increase in total serum bilirubin >85 μmol/L (<u>5</u> mg/dL) per day

c. Total serum bilirubin ><u>200</u> μmol/L (12 mg/dL)

d. Conjugated bilirubin <u>25–35</u> μmol/L (<u>1.5–2</u> mg/dL)

e. Persistence of jaundice for <u>7–10</u> days or <u>2</u> weeks in pre-term babies

8. a–3   b–1   c–4   d–2   e–3   f–2 and
1   g–4   h–2   i–3   j–3   k–1

9. **a.** RhD **incompatibility** can occur when a woman with **Rh-negative** blood type is pregnant with a **Rh-positive fetus**. The placenta acts as a barrier to fetal blood entering the maternal circulation. During pregnancy or birth, fetomaternal haemorrhage (FMH) can occur when small amounts of fetal **Rh-positive** blood cross the placenta and enter the **Rh-negative** mother's blood. The woman's immune system produces **anti-D** antibodies. In subsequent pregnancies these maternal antibodies can cross the placenta and destroy the red cells of any **Rh-positive** fetus.

b. ABO **isoimmunization** usually occurs when the mother is blood **group O** and the baby is blood **group A** (or less often **group B**). Individuals with **type O** blood develop antibodies throughout life from exposure to antigens in food, Gram-**negative** bacteria or blood transfusion. The woman usually has high serum **anti-A** and **anti-B** antibody titres by the time she is pregnant for the first time. Some women produce **IgG** antibodies that can cross the placenta and attach to the red cells and destroy them.

10. True: a, b, d, e, f, g

False: c

ANSWERS

1. True: a, b, e, f, g, i, j, k, m

   False: c, d, h, l

2. a–11   b–6   c–12   d–3   e–6, 7, 8, 9, 13
   f–2   g–4   h–1   i–10   j–5

3.

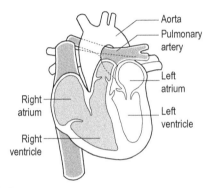

Figure 20.1

4. i. In this condition the aorta arises from the **right** ventricle and the pulmonary artery arises from the **left** ventricle.

   ii. **Oxygenated** blood is circulated back through the lungs and **deoxygenated** blood is circulated back into the systemic circulation.

   iii. A **patent ductus arteriosus** needs to be maintained to provide opportunity for **oxygenated** blood to access the systemic circulation. Otherwise the baby will die.

5.

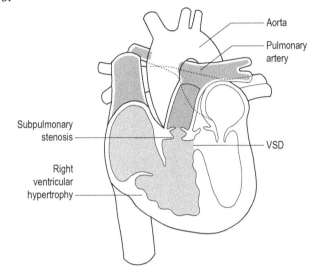

Figure 20.2

6. i. pulmonary outflow is <u>obstructed</u>, ii. ventricular septal defect (VSD), iii. right ventricle is <u>hypertrophied</u>, iv. the aorta is <u>overriding</u>.

7. i. Persistent ductus arteriosus

   ii. Ventricular septal defects

   iii. Atrial septal defects

8. a. <u>tachypnoea</u>   b. <u>tachycardia</u>   c. <u>cyanosis</u>
   d. <u>heart murmurs</u>

9. a. Spina bifida results from <u>failure</u> of fusion of the <u>vertebral column</u>.

   b. A meningocele refers to the protrusion of the <u>meninges</u> through the defect. It does <u>not</u> contain neural tissue.

   c. Meningomyocele refers to the protrusion of <u>meninges</u> through the defect and it involves the <u>spinal cord</u>.

   d. Encephalocele is the term used when the defect is at the <u>level</u> of the <u>base</u> of the skull.

10.

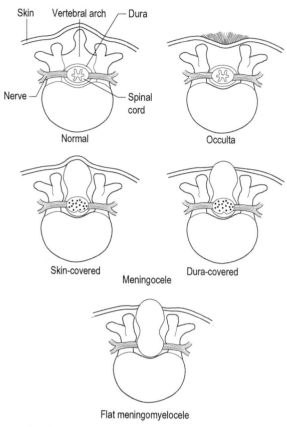

Normal

Occulta

Skin-covered   Dura-covered

Meningocele

Flat meningomyelocele

Figure 20.3

11. a–5   b–1   c–6   d–4   e–2   f–3   g–8   h–7   i–9

12. These infants have **low** blood glucose concentrations because of the excess of **insulin**. This is produced by the fetal **pancreatic gland** as a result of stimulation by **increased** maternal **glucose** concentrations. This excess of **insulin** also acts as a **growth factor** and brings about **excessive** fat and glycogen deposition. The baby usually has a macrosomic appearance.

13. True: b, c, f, g, h, i, j

False: a, d, e